The Psychiatric Drug Handbook

The Psychiatric Drug Handbook

Barry H. Guze, M.D.
Associate Professor
Department of Psychiatry and Biobehavioral Sciences
Department of Radiological Sciences
UCLA School of Medicine
Director
Adult Psychiatry Hospital Service
UCLA Neuropsychiatric Institute and Hospital
Los Angeles, CA

Huan-Kwang Ferng, M.D.
Lecturer, Department of Psychiatry
Tri-Service General Hospital
National Defence Medical Center
Taipei, Taiwan, R.O.C.
Visiting Fellow, Consultation-Liaison
Department of Psychiatry and
Biobehavioral Sciences
UCLA Neuropsychiatric Institute and Hospital
Los Angeles, California

Martin P. Szuba, M.D.
Assistant Professor of Psychiatry
University of Pennsylvania School of Medicine
Philadelphia, PA

Steven H. Richeimer, M.D.
Assistant Professor of Clinical Anesthesiology and Psychiatry
Director
UCD Pain Management Center
University of California at Davis Medical Center
Sacramento, CA

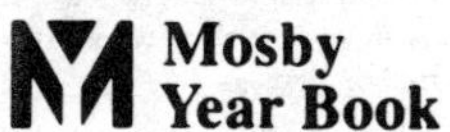

St. Louis Baltimore Boston Chicago London Philadelphia Sydney Toronto

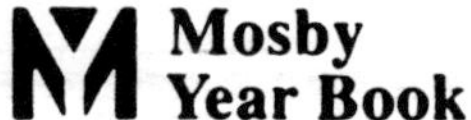

Dedicated to Publishing Excellence

Sponsoring Editor: Nancy Megley
Associate Managing Editor, Manuscript Services: Deborah Thorp
Production Coordinator: Nancy C. Baker
Proofroom Manager: Barbara Kelly

A Year Book Medical Publishers imprint of Mosby-Year Book, Inc.
Mosby-Year Book, Inc., 11830 Westline Industrial Drive, St. Louis, MO 63146

2 3 4 5 6 7 8 9 0 UG/PC 96 95

Library of Congress Cataloging-in-Publication Data

Guze, Barry.
The psychiatric drug handbook/Barry H. Guze, Huan-Kwang Ferng, Martin P. Szuba, Steven Richeimer.
p. cm.
Includes bibliographical references and index.
ISBN 0-8151-4013-4
1. Psychopharmacology—Handbooks, manual, etc. I. Richeimer, Steven. II. Szuba, Martin P. III. Title
[DNLM: 1. Mental Disorders—drug therapy—handbooks. 2. Psychotropic Drugs—therapeutic use—handbooks. WM 34 G993p]
RC483.G89 1991
616.89' 18—dc20
DNLM/DLC 91-31140
for Library of Congress CIP

NOTICE

Every effort has been made to ensure that the drug dosage schedules herein are accurate and in accord with the standards accepted at the time of publication. However, as new research and experience broaden our knowledge, changes in treatment and drug therapy occur. Therefore, the reader is advised to check the product information sheet included in the package of each drug he plans to administer to be certain that changes have not been made in the recommended dose or in the contraindications. This is of particular importance in regard to new or infrequently used drugs.

PREFACE

The *Psychiatric Drug Handbook* was written to provide concise but comprehensive information regarding those pharmaceutical products most frequently used for treating psychiatric disorders. It originated from a need to provide the diverse practitioners who encounter mentally disturbed patients with a concise and readily available source of current drug information.

The scope of drugs reviewed in this work is clear testimony to the continued "medicalization" of psychiatry and advances in the field, reflecting the increasing amount of medical information necessary to treat psychiatric patients effectively. We hope this book will prove useful not only to active practitioners of clinical psychiatry and psychiatric trainees, but also to general practitioners, family practitioners, nurses, and other health care providers involved in treating mentally ill patients. Particularly for practitioners, it will serve as a ready source of information about commonly available preparations of psychotropic drugs, and as a ready resource for reviewing indications, contraindications, and common side effects associated with the use of these agents.

In Chapter 1, the introduction, we review the fundamental principles which we believe should govern the use of psychotropic drugs. For the remainder of the book, drugs are grouped into chapters according to their common pharmacologic properties. Each chapter opens with a description of the features shared by the particular class of agents, then is subdivided into discussions of individual drugs. For each, specific details are provided including the usual dosage and available preparations.

The *Psychiatric Drug Handbook* is not intended as an introductory textbook to the clinical use of psychopharmacologic agents. Rather, it is best utilized as a handy reference to be consulted frequently as practical clinical problems arise. Psychiatrists and primary care physicians responsible for treating those complex individuals who suffer from cognitive disturbances, emotional difficulties, behavioral disorders, addictions, and dependencies can rely on this work as an up-to-date source of fundamental pharmacologic information to aid them in their daily practice.

Barry H. Guze, M.D.
Huan-Kwang Ferng, M.D.
Martin P. Szuba, M.D.
Steven Richeimer, M.D.

ACKNOWLEDGMENT

Writing a book is a major endeavor. It requires organization, motivation, and persistence. Phyllis Davis has repeatedly demonstrated not only these traits, but also patience and good humor. Without her, this book would not exist.

The authors join to thank her, with affection, for her outstanding efforts.

Barry H. Guze, M.D.
Huan-Kwang Ferng, M.D.
Martin P. Szuba, M.D.
Steven Richeimer, M.D.

CONTENTS

INTRODUCTION OVERVIEW OF PSYCHO-PHARMACOLOGY 1

Psychopharmacology is not an exact science. Indeed, much of our knowledge is empirical. Usually medications are used to alleviate rather than cure disease. Nevertheless, psychoactive medications provide patients with levels of relief undreamed of less than half a century ago. New and better drugs are being developed rapidly. Many of these drugs are reviewed in later chapters; this introductory chapter, organized by diagnosis, is aimed at providing an overview of treatment. Detailed pharmacologic information about each medication is provided in subsequent chapters.

AFFECTIVE DISORDERS

Major Depression

The majority of all psychiatric prescriptions are for depressive disorders. One in five Americans will suffer from a major depression at some time during his or her life. Various anti-depressant medications are helpful in the treatment of this illness (Table 1–1).

Serotonin reuptake inhibitors are the primary drugs used in the treatment of depression. The tricyclic and heterocyclic antidepressants (Table 1–2) have been used extensively in the past because the efficacy of these drugs has extensive support in the scientific literature and clinical experience. However, a number of problems exist with these drugs (Table 1–3). The tricyclics have many side effects that are troublesome or outright dangerous in some patients. Patients with cardiac conduction distutbances, prostatic hypertrophy, or narrow-angle glaucoma, or the elderly, may be unable to safely tolerate these medications. Tricyclics are potentially lethal in overdose; therefore, they may be difficult to administer to patients with strong suicidal impulses. For many otherwise healthy patients, the anticholinergic side effects or possible weight gain may be intolerable.

The monoamine oxidase inhibitors (MAOIs) have also been a mainstay in the treatment of depression. Traditionally, these medi-

Table 1–1.
Major Selection Criteria for Use of Antidepressants in Mood Disorders*†

Drug	Initial Amine(s) Affected	Sedative/ Stimulant Activity‡	Anticholinergic Activity	Orthostatic Hypotension	Cardiac Toxicity	Seizure Gain	Weight Gain	Comments
Tricyclic antidepressants Amitriptyline (Elavil)	5-HT++ NE± DA0	↓↓	+++	++	+++	++	++	
Amoxapine (Asendin)	5-HT NE++ DA0	↓	+	+	++	++	+/0	Infrequently, extrapyramidal reactions develop. A relatively high incidence of seizures occurs in patients who have taken excessive amounts.
Desipramine (Norpramin, Pertrofrane)	5-H0 NE+++ DA0	↓	+	+	++	+	+	
Doxepine (Adapin, Sinequan)	5-HT NE+ DA0	↓↓↓	+++	+	++	++	+	
Imipramine (Janimine, Tofranil)	5-HT+ NE+ DA0	↓↓	++	++	+++	++	+	

Maprotiline (Ludiomil)	5-HT0 NE++ DA0	↓↓	++	+	++	+++	+	Incidence of skin rash is 3%. Incidence of seizures is highest among the tricyclic compounds, which are pharmacologically quite similar to maprotiline, a tetracyclic compound.
Nortriptyline (Aventyl, Pamelor)	5-HT± NE++ DA0	↓↓	+	±	++	++	+	
Protriptyline (Vivactil)	5-HT+ NE++ DA0	↓	++	+	+++	++	+	
Trimipramine (Surmontil)	5-HT+++ NE+	↓↓↓	++	++	+++	++	+	
Atypical antidepressants[§] Bupropion (Wellbutrin)	5-HT± NE± DA++	↑	0	0	0	++++	0/–	Incidence of seizures is fourfold higher than with the tricyclic compounds when recommended dose ranges are exceeded. Preferable dose is ≤ 300 mg/day; maximum is 450 mg/day. Extrapyramidal reactions and worsening of psychoses have been observed infrequently.
Fluoxetine (Prozac)	5-HT+++ NE0 DA0	↑	0	0	±	+	0/–	

(Continued)

Table 1–1 (cont.).

Drug	Initial Amine(s) Affected	Sedative/ Stimulant Activity‡	Anticholinergic Activity	Orthostatic Hypotension	Cardiac Toxicity	Seizure Gain	Weight Gain	Comments
Trazodone (Deseyrel)	5-HT+ NE0 DA0	↓↓	±	+	++	+	+/0	Prolonged priapism may occur (incidence, 1:6,000) within 1–2 weeks after initiating therapy; medical intervention may be required.
Alprazolam (Xanax)	5-HT0 NE0 DA0	↓↓↓	0	0	0	0	0	Dependence and withdrawl reactions usually occur on abrupt discontinuation of this drug following prolonged therapy (weeks), especially with the larger doses required for treatment of mood disorders. Efficacy in severe major depression has not been established.
Monoamine oxidase	5-HT++	↓	0	++	0	0	+	

Inhibitors (MAOIs) Isocarboxazid (Marplan)	NE++ DA++							Food and MAOI interactions require education of the patient and vigilant monitoring by the physician to minimize toxicity.
Phenelzine (Nardil)	5-HT++ NE++ DA++	↓	0	++	0	0	±	
Tranylcypromine (Parnate)	5-HT++ NE++ DA++	↑	0	++	0	0	+/0	

* Adapted from *The American Medical Association Drug Evaluations Book.* Chicago, American Medical Association, 1990.

† 5-HT = serotonin; NE = norepinephrine; DA = dopamine; 0 = none; + = mild; ++ = moderate; +++ = marked; ++++ = severe; ± = equivocal; − = weight loss.

‡ Sedative activity is indicated by ↓ and stimulant activity by ↑. The number of symbols represents a relative estimate of the intensity of the effect within columns, but does not reflect the absolute incidence of side effects across columns.

§ Alternative designations for the atypical depressants in various publications are second-generation; "newer"; or selective neurotransmitter amine reuptake inhibitors or agonist antidepressants or both, to differentiate them from the tricyclic and MAOI classes of antidepressants.

Table 1–2.
Antidepressant Drugs and Their Approximate Effective Dose Ranges*

Generic Name	Effective Dose Range (mg/day)
Imipramine	150–300
Amitriptyline	150–250
Desipramine	75–200g
Nortriptyline	30–100
Protriptyline	15–40
Doxepin	75–300
Tricyclic-type drugs	
Trimipramine	75–300
Maprotiline	75–150
Amoxapine	50–300
Monoamine oxidase	
Tranylcypromine	20–60
Isocarboxazid	20–60
Phenelzine	60–60

*Adapted from Kaplan HI, Sadock BJ (eds): *Modern Synopsis of the Comprehensive Textbook of Psychiatry,* ed 4. Baltimore, Williams & Wilkins, p. 656.

cations have been used as second-line treatment if the patient has failed to respond to tricyclics, or as first-line treatment for atypical depressions (characterized by high levels of anxiety, neuroticism, overeating, and oversleeping). The primary problem with this group of drugs is that acute hypertensive crises can occur if the patient consumes foods high in tyramine or ingests sympathomimetic or some narcotic medications (Table 1–4). Therefore, the patient must be carefully instructed with regard to diet and the avoidance of all new medications (including over-the-counter remedies) without checking with his or her physician. Furthermore, these drugs have other potential side effects that may limit their usefulness: orthostatic hypotension, sedation or insomnia, sexual dysfunction, and weight gain. These medications are also potentially lethal in overdose.

Fortunately, in recent years, other antidepressant medications have been added to the psychiatric armamentarium. These include trazodone, fluoxetine, and bupropion. These drugs all present less hazard in situations of overdose, and have fewer side effects (especially anticholinergic effects). Importantly, fluoxetine and bupropion are not associated with weight gain or sedation.

Stimulants, most commonly methylphenidate, are also useful. These are usually second-line or third-line (occasionally first-line)

Table 1–3.
Side Effects of Antidepressant Agents

Aggravation of narrow-angle glaucoma
Agitation
Blurred vision
Constipation
Dry mouth
Edema
Galactorrhea
Heart block
Paralytic ileus
Orthostatic hypotension
Sedation
Urinary retention

drugs in the treatment of depression in the elderly, postcerebral infarct patients, or patients with acquired immunodeficiency syndrome (AIDS). Stimulants are also sometimes used in conjunction with tricyclics, either to help reduce the time preceding an antidepressant medication response, or as an adjunct for patients with refractory depression.

If patients demonstrate psychotic symptoms during a depression, it is important to also administer neuroleptic medication. In this setting, providing antidepressant drugs without neuroleptics may decrease the probability of a successful outcome. In many cases, electroconvulsive therapy (ECT) is the treatment of choice for major depression with psychotic symptoms.

Approximately 70% of patients will respond to treatment with an antidepressant. There is no set protocol for the treatment of the 30% who do not initially respond. The following order of treatments is a rough guideline:

1. Six-weeks of treatment with a tricyclic antidepressant at the maximum (or maximum tolerated) dose. Check serum levels, if available, to insure that adequate doses are being taken and absorbed.

2. Six- to 8 weeks of treatment with a newer antidepressant, e.g., fluoxetine, or bupropion. (In many circumstances, steps 1 and 2 may be reversed.)

3. Three- to 4 weeks of the addition of lithium to the antidepressant currently being tried.

4. Six- to 8 weeks' trial of treatment with an MAOI. Adding an MAOI to existing treatment with tricyclics may be considered; however, tricyclics should not be added to existing treatment with MAOIs. In addition, MAOIs should not be used in conjunction with (or within 5 weeks of) the use of fluoxetine or buproprion.

Table 1–4.
Dietary and Medication Precautions for Patients Taking Monoamine Oxidase Inhibitor (MAO) Antidepressants

Foods That Must Be Avoided	Foods That May Be Consumed With Caution*
Cheese (cottage cheese and cream cheese are safe)	Avocado
Smoked or pickled meats, fish or poultry, caviar; game	Raspberries
Nonfresh meat, nonfresh livers (fresh-frozen meat, liver, poultry, and fish are safe.)	Soy sauce
Chianti and vermouth wines	Chocolate
Distilled spirits to which red wine has been added	Red and white wines (except Chianti and vermouth)
Broad bean pods (fava or Italian broad beans; Chinese pea pods) (string beans, lima beans and dry beans are safe)	Port, sherry
Banana peel	Distilled spirits
Meat extracts used as a base for soup, gravy and sauces (bouillon, consommé, Bovril)	Yogurt from unpasteurized milk
Sausage, corned beef (bacon is safe)	Cream from unpasteurized milk
Sauerkraut	
Beer, ale, etc., wiith or without alcohol	Miso soup or soup stock

Any food, especially a high-protein food, should not be used unless freshly prepared with brief shelf storage. Do not consume any food that previously caused illness or unpleasant symptoms.

Medications That Must Be Avoided

Medications or preparations (tablets, capsules, drops, sprays, and inhalants) for colds, nasal, sinus, or throat congestion, coughs, hay fever, nasal, or sinus allergy, or asthma

Medications or preparations for weight reduction or appetite control or suppression

Demerol (meperidine)

Dextromethorphan (often used as cough suppressant)

Cocaine, amphetamines, "uppers," or "pep pills"

Epinephrine (often added to local anesthetics as for dental procedures)

Other antidepresssants unless approved by your doctor

Do not take any medications, drugs or proprietary preparations of any kind without first consulting your doctor

Follow these food and medication precautions and carry them with you throughout the time that you are taking the MAOI and continue, to do so for two weeks after stopping the MAOI.

*Consumed with caution: small servings (1/2 cup, 4 oz, 120 mL or less).

Table 1–5.
Method of Predicting Initial Dosage Regimen of Lithium Therapy*

Procedure:

The patient is given a loading dose of lithium carbonate, 600 mg by mouth (po), at 8 A.M. on day 1. Precisely at 8 A.M. (or exactly 24 hr following the loading dose) on day 2, blood is drawn and a serum lithium determination made. The morning dose of lithium must be held until blood is drawn. The resulting serum lithium value is entered into the table below to predict the dosage regimen.

Determination of dosage regimen:

Serum Lithium, mEq/L (24 hr Following 600-mg Loading Dose)	Dosage Regimen to Maintain 0.6–1.2-mEq/L Lithium Level
0.24–0.30†	300 mg BID
0.20–0.23	300 mg TID
0.15–0.19	300 mg QID
0.10–0.14	600 mg TID
0.05–0.09	900 mg TID
0.05	1200 mg TID

*Adapted from Cooper TB, Simpson GM: *Am J Psychiatry* 1978; 133:440–443.
†For serum levels above 0.30 mEq/L, lithium should be administrated with caution, and further patient evaluation is advised.

5. Consider treatment with ECT. ECT might be considered a first-line treatment for patients with psychotic depression, intense suicidality, or frail patients who might not be able to tolerate medication.

or

Consider more novel antidepressant treatments: buspirone (there are reports of antidepressant efficacy), phototherapy, thyroid hormone supplementation, or stimulants (either as solo treatment or as supplementation). In the elderly, stimulants may be considered much earlier in the treatment hierarchy.

Bipolar Disorder

This disorder is characterized by episodes of depression and episodes of mania. Depressed patients must have a history of at least one previous episode of mania in order to receive a diagnosis of bipolar disorder, rather than major depression. Any patient with a history of mania (whether or not he or she previously had a depressive episode) is diagnosed as having bipolar disorder.

The first-line treatment of this disorder is lithium (Table 1–5). This medication has proved highly effective in the treatment of

Table 1–6.
Possible Effects of Lithium on Laboratory Values*

Laboratory Values	Possible Effect of Lithium
White blood cell count	Increased
Serum glucose	Increased
Serum magnesium	Increased
Serum potassium	Decreased
Serum uric acid	Decreased
Serum thyroxine	Decreased
Serum cortisol	Decreased A.M. levels
Serum parathyroid hormone	Increased due to adenoma
Serum calcium	Increased due to increased parathyroid hormone level
Serum phosphorus	Decreased due to increased parathyroid hormone level

*Adapted from Guze BH (ed): *The Handbook of Psychiatry.* Chicago, Year Book, 1990, p 386.

bipolar episodes of mania or depression; it is also effective in the prophylaxis of further episodes. During the acute treatment of mania, neuroleptics are usually administered concurrently with lithium. If the level of agitation is severe, additional sedation with benzodiazepines, e.g., parenteral lorazepam, or neuroleptics may be necessary.

Lithium may produce a variety of laboratory abnormalities (Table 1–6). It may also produce various side effects (Table 1–7). In addition, lithium may pose a significant risk in some conditions (Table 1–8).

Treatment of bipolar depression is often successful with lithium; if, however, the depression persists or is severe, antidepressant medications are often added. In 7% to 17% of patients, antidepressant medication can precipitate a switch from depression into mania. Buproprion may be less likely to precipitate such a switch. If the depression is complicated with a psychosis, then neuroleptics are often also administered.

If lithium does not effectively prevent or treat affective episodes, then carbamazepine can be used, either alone or added to lithium. Many clinicians consider carbamazepine to be the treatment of choice for rapid cycling bipolar disorder. Carbamazepine also has a variety of significant side effects. Some of these may be-come severe enough to indicate drug discontinuation (Table 1–9). If a poor response or side effects limit the use of

Table 1–7.
Side Effects of Lithium and Their Management*

Side Effect	Management
Gastrointestinal complaints	Give lithium after meals; give smaller doses more often; try slow-release preparation; lower the dose
Tremor complaints	Lower the dose; give propranolol (40–100 mg/day); consider adding a benzodiazepine
Polyuria/diabetes insipidus	Try slow-release preparation; lower the dose; add amiloride (5–10 mg/day); carefully monitor lithium levels
Acne	Benzoyl peroxide (5%–10% topical solution, erythromycin (1.5%–2.0%) topical solutio
Muscular weakness, fasciculations, headaches	Usually resolve with first few weeks of treatment
Hypothyroidism	Levothyroxine (0.05 mg/day), follow thyroid-stimulating hormone level and increase to 0.2 mg/day as needed
T wave inversion	Benign; no treatment needed
Cardiac dysrhythmias	Usually must discontinue lithium
Psoriasis, alopecia areata	Dermatology consult; reversible if lithium stopped
Weight gain	Difficult to treat; diet; may be partially reversible if lithium stopped
Edema	Consider spironolactone (50 mg/day po); if severe, monitor lithium levels; resolves when lithium stopped
Leukocytosis	Benign, no treatment needed

*Adapted from Guze BH (ed): *The Handbook of Psychiatry.* Chicago, Year Book, 1990, p 386.

lithium or carbamazepine, then third-line treatments need to be considered. These include valproate, ECT, and adjunctive treatment with clonazepam.

Cyclothymia

The effectiveness of pharmacologic treatment of this disorder is controversial. Lithium or carbamazepine are the drugs generally used. Some clinicians believe that cyclothymia frequently progresses into bipolar disorder, and that treatment may prevent this development.

Dysthymia

The effectiveness of pharmacologic treatment of this disorder is also controversial. Any of the antidepressant medications may be tried; some clinicians believe that MAOIs or fluoxetine may be more effective than other antidepressants.

Table 1–8.
Conditions in Which Lithium Use Poses Significant Risk*

Condition	Potential Problem	Management Approach
Pregnancy (especially 1st trimester)	Increased risk of fetus developing tetralogy of Fallot	Avoid lithium in 1st trimester; electro convulsive therapy or neuroleptics are safer; general counseling; consider abortion if lithium used
Breast-feeding	Lithium toxicity from lithium excreted in breast milk	No breast-feeding with lithium; provide formula feeding
Sick sinus syndrome	Cardiac arrest reported tetralogy of Fallot	Consider pacemaker placement, ECT, neuroleptics
Postmyocardial infarction Altered fluid and electrolyte status	Potential for dysrhythmias Potential for lithium toxicity	Slow dose increases; frequent ECG monitoring; hold lithium and consider neuroleptics
Labor and delivery	Lithium toxicity in mother due to fluid shifts; lithium toxicity in infant	Reduce dose by 50% in last week of pregnancy; discontinue lithium at onset of labor
Renal insufficiency	Delayed excretion increases half-life and increases risk of developing toxic levels	Reduce dosage
Advanced age	Side effects and therapeutic response often at lower doses; increased serum levels at usual therapeutic doses secondary to diminished renal function	Initiate treatment at a low dosage; increase gradually
Organic brain syndromes	Side effects, especially cognitive changes, are more likely	Low initial dosages, gradual increases

*Adapted from Guze BH (ed): *The Handbook of Psychiatry*. Chicago, Year Book Medical Publishers, 1989, p 382.

Table 1–9.
Guidelines for Discontinuing Carbamazepine Therapy*

Indicator	Value
WBC count	<3,000/mm^3
Neutrophils	<1,500/mm^3
Erythrocytes	<4.0 x 10^6/mm^3
Hematocrit	<32%
Hemoglobin level	11 g/100 mL
Platelet count	100,000/mm^3
Reticulocyte count	<0.3%
Serum iron level	150 mg/100 mL

*Adapted from Guze BH (ed): *The Handbook of Psychiatry*. Chicago, Year Book, 1990, p 393.

SCHIZOPHRENIA AND NONAFFECTIVE PSYCHOSES

Psychosis is characterized by delusions, hallucinations, incoherence of thought processes, or grossly disorganized behavior. The prototypical psychotic illness is schizophrenia; however, psychosis also occurs with affective and other disorders. Other nonaffective psychoses include brief reactive psychosis, atypical psychosis, delirium, delusional disorder, and postpartum psychosis.

The neuroleptics are the primary treatment for psychotic symptoms (Table 1–10). If there is an underlying, treatable cause, e.g., delirium secondary to septicemia, then this must also be treated. The neuroleptics are all of approximately equal efficacy; the choice of drug is usually determined by its side effect profile (Table 1–11, 1–12, 1–13, 1–14). Generally, the low-potency neuroleptics are more sedating, have more anticholinergic effects, and produce more orthostatic hypotension. The high-potency neuroleptics have more extrapyramidal side effects, including akathisia. The presence of extrapyramidal side effects may require the coadministration of anticholinergic or dopaminergic (e.g., amantadine) medications (Table 1–15). β-blockers or benzodiazepines may be useful for the treatment of akathisia. The prolonged administration of any of the neuroleptics is associated with a 15% to 20% risk of developing tardive dyskinesia.

Neuroleptics are used both for the treatment of acute agitation in the psychotic patient, and for the long-term treatment of the psychotic symptoms. The combined use of high-potency neuroleptics and intramuscular (IM) lorazepam (e.g., haloperidol 5 mg IM, lorazepam 2 mg IM) for the treatment of severe agitation has recently been advocated by some. The addition of the benzodiazepine provides sedation, allowing the patient's symptoms to be controlled without the increased risk of unpleasant or dangerous side effects that are sometimes associated with high doses of neuroleptics.

Schizophrenia

As with other psychoses, the first-line treatment for schizophrenia is neuroleptic medication. Schizophrenic patients usually require long-term treatment. There is considerable controversy in the clinical literature regarding the appropriate dose for a maintenance neuroleptic. The dilemma is that higher doses over prolonged time periods are associated with poorer compliance and a greater risk of tardive dyskinesia; however, low doses are associated with higher rates of relapse. Decisions regarding the maintenance dose of a neuroleptic medication should be made on a case-by-case basis.

Some patients may not respond well to neuroleptics, or may be unable to tolerate the side effects. A new antipsychotic medication, clozapine, is available for those patients who have not responded adequately to several prior trials of conventional neuroleptics. The primary problem with this medication is a relatively high risk of development of agranulocytosis. Patients receiving this medication must have their complete blood cell count checked weekly.

ALCOHOL ABUSE

Alcohol abuse is associated with a wide variety of syndromes that may require psychiatric treatment. Withdrawal syndromes may range from mild discomfort to seizures, delirium, and even death. Symptoms of alcohol withdrawal syndrome usually begin within 12 hours after cessation of heavy drinking. Initially there is tremulousness, which may be followed by autonomic hyperactivity, insomnia, nightmares, and acute anxiety.

Ten percent of patients with alcohol withdrawal will experience withdrawal seizures. These usually occur between 8 and 48 hours after cessation of drinking.

The most severe form of alcohol withdrawal is delirium tremens. This usually occurs on the third or fourth day of abstinence. Approximately 5% of hospitalized alcoholics will suffer with delirium tremens. The primary symptoms are tremor, autonomic hyperactivity and instability, and delirium with disturbed sleep-wake cycle, impaired cognitive processing (including confusion and disorientation), and perceptual disturbance (illusions or hallucinations). These patients are often very frightened and they may act in unpredictable and potentially dangerous ways.

The basic pharmacologic treatment for all of the alcohol withdrawal syndromes is gradual detoxification with a cross-reacting sedative drug. Barbiturates can be used for this purpose; however, it is safer to use long-acting benzodiazepines, such as chlordiazepoxide or diazepam (Table 1–16). Treatment of the initial and milder symptoms may help prevent the development of the more severe, later syndromes. Treatment should be titrated to the point at which symptoms are subsiding rather than progressing. Typically, during the initial syndrome, patients will require 25 to 50 mg of chlordiazepoxide every 3 to 6 hours (or 5–10 mg of diazepam every 3–6 hours). If delirium develops, then patients typically require 50 to 100 mg of chlordiazepoxide (orally, IM, or intravenously [IV]) every 4 hours. Absorption of IM diazepam or chlordiazepoxide may be erratic. Occasionally, to control the initial agitation and autonomic instability of delirium tremens, patients may require 50 to 100 mg/ry hr; more than 500 mg should not be given during a 24-hour period. Alternatively, 5 mg of diazepam may be given by slow IV push (5 mg/min), and repeated every 5 to 15 minutes until the patient becomes calm; do not exceed 20 mg of diazepam in the first hour, or 60 mg/24 hr. Once the patient's condition has stabilized and he or she is out of danger, then the daily dose of benzodiazepine should be reduced by 25%-50% per day, as tolerated by the patient.

For patients with hepatic insufficiency, benzodiazepines that only require metabolic conjugation, e.g., lorazepam or oxazepam, are preferable.

Correction of the nutritional deficiencies associated with alcoholism and delirium tremens is important. Thiamine, 100 mg IV is given prior to any IV glucose solution; 100 mg/day is subsequently administered. Magnesium sulfate, 1 g/day, IV (or if the patient has not developed delirium tremens, a one-time dose of magnesium sulfate, 1 cc IM in each buttock) is sufficient to treat hypomagnesemia and decrease the risk of seizures.

Hallucinations may occur during alcohol withdrawal. If they do not respond to treatment with benzodiazepines, then a high-potency neuroleptic may be helpful (e.g., haloperidol, 5 mg every 2–4 hours), until symptoms subside or a maximum of 20 mg is reached.

Table 1–10.
Neuroleptic Medications: Potency and Dosages*†

Chemical Group, Generic Name (Trade Name)	Relative Potency	Approximate Equivalent Dose (mg/day)	Usual Adult Dosages	
			Oral (mg/day)	Single IM
Phenothiazines				
Aliphatic				
Chlorpromazine (Thorazine) (g)	Low	100	100–1,500	25–100
Piperidine				
Mesoridazine (Serentil)	Low	50	50–400	25
Thioridazine (Mellaril) (g)	Low	100	100–800	NA
Piperazine				
Fluphenazine (Prolixin, Permitil)	High	2–3	2–20	1.25–2.5 (of HCl)
Trifluoperazine (Stelazine) (g)	High	3–5	5–50	1–2
Perphenazine (Trilafon)	Medium	5–10	8–65	5–10
Thioxanthenes				
Chlorprothixene (Taractan)	Low	100	75–600	25–50
Thiothixene (Navane)	High	3–5	5–60	2–6

Butyrophenones				
Haloperidol (Haldol)	High	2–3	2–20	2.5–5.0
Droperidol (Inapsine)	High	1–2	NA	5–10 IM 5–100 IV
Dihydroindolones				
Molindone (Moban)	Medium	10	50–225	NA
Dibenzoxapines				
Loxapine (Loxitane)	Medium	10–15	50–250	12.5–25
Diphenylbutyl-piperidines				
Pimozide (Orap)	High	1–2	1–20	NA

*Adapted from Baldessarini RJ: *Chemotherapy in Psychiatry*. Cambridge, Mass, Harvard University Press, 1985; and Mason AS, Granacher RP: *Clinical Handbook of Anti-Psychotic Drug Therapy*. New York, Brunner/Mazel, 1980.

†(g) = generic form available; NA = not available.

Table 1–11.
Neuroleptic Medications: Side Effect Profiles*†

Generic Name	Anticholinergic	Extrapyramidal	Hypotension	Sedation
Chlorpromazine	+ + +	+ + +	Oral + + IM + +	+ +
Mesoridazine	+ +	+ +	+ +	+ + +
Thioridazine	+ + +	+ +	+ +	+
Fluphenazine	+	+	+	+ + +
Trifluoperazine	+	+	+	+ +
Perphenazine	+	+	+	+ +
Chlorprothixene	+ + +	+ +	+ +	+ +
Thiothixene	+	+	+	+ + +
Haloperidol	+	+	+	+ + +
Droperidol	+ + +	+	±	+
Molindone	+ +	+ +	0	+
Loxapine	+ +	+ +	+	+ +
Pimozide	+	+	±	+ + +

*Adapted from Baldessarini RJ: *Chemotherapy in Psychiatry: Principles and Practice.* Cambridge, Mass, Harvard University Press, 1985.
† 0 = rare; + = mild; + + = marked; + + + = severe; ± = equivocal.

Table 1–12.
Peripheral Side Effects of Neuroleptic Medications*

Body System	Clinical Feature	Proposed Mechanism	Treatment	Common Offenders and Commens
Automatic nervous system				
A. Cardiovascular	Dizziness, postural hypotension	α-adrenergic blockade	Decrease dose; support hose	Thorazine, thioridazine
B. Gastrointestinal	Dry mouth, constipation	Anticholinergic	Decrease dose; decrease concomitant anti-cholinergics, stool softeners	Thorazine, Mellaril
C. Genitourinary	Urinary hesistancy, retention; absent, delayed, retrograde ejaculation delayed, retrograde),	Anticholinergic; multiple autonomic effects	Decrease dose; decrease or stop concomitant anti-cholinergic medications	Low-potency agents >
D. Vision	Blurred vision	Anticholinergic	Decrease anti-cholinergic agents; pilo-carpine eye drops	Tolerance usually develops

(Continued.)

Table 1–12. (cont.).

Body System	Clinical Featuresk	Proposed Mechanism	Treatment	Common Offenders and Commens
Ophthalmologic	Precipitation of narrow-angle glaucoma	Anticholinergic	Immediate medical treatment	
	Pigmentary retinopathy	Drug-melanin interaction in retina	Avoid > 800 mg thioridazine	Thioridazine
Cardiac	ECG effects; ST segment depression, T wave flattening, increased PR, QRS, and/or QT interval	Quinidine-like effect	Discontinue medication if clinically indicated	Low-potency agents, especially thioridazine; clinical significance of ECG changes uncertain
		Anticholinergic	Decrease or stop anticholinegics	
Allergic				
A. Dermatoses	Urticarial, maculopapular	Drug-protein complexes in skin	Stop medication	Phenothiazines, especially chlorpromazine
Systematic photosensitivity	Severe sunburn	Allergic	Prevent by using sunscreens	Phenothiazines

B. Agranulocytosis	Unexplained sore throat, fever, malaise	Unknown	Stop medication; reverse isolation; antibiotics; supportive care	Chlorpromazine
Leukopenia	Lowered WBC count	Unknown	Benign; usually is transient	Low-potency agents
C. Hepatotoxicity, jaundice, elevated liver enzymes	Jaundice followed in 1–7 days by fever, nausea, right upper quadrant pain, malaise	Idiosyncratic	Stop drug	Low-potency agents
Metabolic and endocrine	Galactorrhea, irregular menses or amenorrhea; gynecomastia	Prolactin elevation	In females rule out pregnancy; decrease dose	All agents
	Decreased libido	Hypothalamic	Decrease dose	May be > with thioridazine in men
	Polydipsia, edema	Inappropriate ADH secretion	Rule out SIADH	
	Weight gain	? Hypothalamic	Restrict caloric intake; increase exercise; decrease dose	Most with low-potency agents, least with molindone

*Adapted from Baldessarini RJ: *Chemotherapy in Psychiatry: Principles and Practice*. Cambridge, Mass, Harvard Univversity Press, 1985; and Lydiard RB, et al in Gold MS, et al (eds): *Advances in Psychopharmacology*. Boca Raton, Fla, CRC Press, 1984.

Wernicke-Korsakoff (Alcohol Amnestic) Syndrome

Prolonged alcohol abuse may lead to the development of the alcohol amnestic syndrome, which is characterized by severe short-term memory disturbance, but without impairment of immediate recall. The chronic stage of this syndrome is known as Korsakoff's dementia or psychosis, and is irreversible. However, this chronic stage may be preceded by an acute Wernicke's encephalopathy. The characteristic signs of this syndrome are ataxia, ophthalmoplegia, nystagmus, and confusion. The latter syndrome should be immediately treated with thiamine 50 mg IM or 50 mg IV, followed by 100 mg orally daily.

In the emergency treatment of altered mental status of unknown cause, parenteral thiamine should be administered before IV glucose or other carbohydrate loads are given. Thiamine is a cofactor in glucose metabolism; a sudden glucose load may deplete low thiamine stores, and precipitate Wernicke's encephalopathy.

ORGANIC BRAIN SYNDROMES

The organic brain syndromes are classified as either dementias or deliria. Dementia is characterized by a deficit in intellectual functioning, including language, memory, calculations, judgment, and abstraction. Changes in personality and visuospatial skills are also found. Generally, the onset is gradual, and the course of the symptoms is chronic.

Delirium is characterized by impaired or fluctuating alertness with impairments in cognitive processing, thought content, perception, mood, and the sleep-wake cycle. There may also be disturbances in autonomic functioning (e.g., fluctuating vital signs, flushing, constipation, or diarrhea) and motor system functioning (e.g., tremor, myoclonus, dysarthria, or hyperactivity). The onset of delirium is often rapid, and the course of the syndrome is fluctuating and usually short (hours or days).

Treatment of organic brain syndromes rests primarily on treating the underlying cause of the brain dysfunction. Unfortunately, for many of the dementias this is not possible. For both dementia and delirium it is essential to identify potentially reversible etiologies. Almost all categories of medical illness can be associated with impaired brain function, including toxic, drug withdrawal, infectious (central nervous systen [CNS] or systemic), hormonal,

Table 1–13.
Extrapyramidal and Parkinsonian Side Effects of Neuroleptic Medications*†

Reaction	Features	Period of Maximum Risk	Proposed Mechanism	Treatment
Acute dystonia	Spasm of muscles of tongue, face, neck, and back; may mimic seizures; is not hysteria	1–5 days	Dopamine excess?; acetylcholine excess?	Antiparkinsonian agents are diagnostic and curative (IM or IV, then po)
Parkinsonism	Bradykinesia, rigidity, variable tremor, masklike facies, shuffling gait, dysphagia	5–30 days (may persist)	Dopamine blockade	Antiparkinsonian drugs; try low-potency drug; dopamine agonists risky?
Akathisia	Motor restlessness; patient may experience anxiety or agitation	5–60 days (commonly persists)	Unknown	Lower dose; try low-potency drug; low-dose propranolol; antiparkinsonian agents or benzodiazepines may help
"Rabbit" syndrome	Perioral tremor (late parkinsonism variant?); usually reversible	Month–years	Unknown	Antiparkinsonian agents; reduce dose of neuroleptic
Akinesia (akinetic mutism)	Waxy flexibility, poverty of speech and movement, posturing; sometimes mistaken for true catatonia and treated inappropriately with increase of antipsychotics	1–4 wk	Unknown	Reduce dosage of antiparkinsonian agent

*Adapted from Baldessarini RJ: *Chemotherapy in Psychiatry: Principles and Practice.* Cambridge, Mass, Harvard University Press, 1985.
†Antiparkinsonian agents are presented elsewhere and are typically anticholinergics.

structural (e.g., hydrocephalus), metabolic, nutritional, genetic, vascular, immunologic, neoplastic, degenerative, or traumatic.

In addition to addressing the underlying cause, it may also be necessary to treat symptoms of agitation or psychosis. Low doses of a high-potency neuroleptic (e.g., 1 mg of haloperidol or thiothixene, one to two times per day) may provide some relief. Occasionally, low doses of a readily metabolized benzodiazepine (e.g., lorazepam 0.5 mg, one to two times per day) are used if symptoms of agitation and insomnia are present without psychotic symptoms. The cardinal rule is to keep the doses low. Brain function in these patients has already been disturbed; even the usual doses of benzodiazepines may exacerbate the dysfunction.

ANXIETY DISORDERS

Anxiety disorders affect more than 7% of the US population. Benzodiazepines are the most commonly prescribed group of drugs in the United States which hints at the frequency of anxiety or sleep-related complaints.

Generalized Anxiety Disorder

This disorder is characterized by persistent anxiety of at least 6 months' duration. Symptoms may include apprehension, motor tension, hypervigilance, and autonomic hyperactivity. Traditionally, benzodiazepines have been the drugs of choice for the treatment of this disorder (see Table 1–16). However, buspirone is a relatively new agent of comparable efficacy. Buspirone has significant advantages which often indicate that this drug should be tried before the benzodiazepines. The advantages include less sedation, less interaction with other CNS depressants or alcohol, and no apparent abuse potential or development of dependence. The primary disadvantage of buspirone is its slow onset of action which may be as long as 3 weeks. For this reason it may be necessary in some severely anxious patients to simultaneously administer a benzodiazepine while waiting until the buspirone becomes effective.

It should be noted that anxiety symptoms often respond to treatment with antidepressants (see Table 1–2). In some cases the anxiety may be a symptom of depression or part of a depressive prodrome.

Panic Disorder

Panic disorder is characterized by spontaneous, recurrent attacks of overwhelming anxiety or terror with associated autonomic symptoms. Antidepressants have proved very effective in the treatment of this disorder—the most commonly studied antidepressants for this purpose are imipramine and phenelzine (see Table 1–2). Patients with this disorder often appear to be hypersensitive to or hyperaware of unusual somatic sensations, and therefore often react negatively to the side effects of these drugs. It is prudent to initiate treatment with smaller-than-usual antidepressant doses, and to increase the dosage more slowly.

Alprazolam is also effective in the short-term treatment of panic disorder. The treatment of panic may require higher doses than typically used for anxiety disorder. The primary problems with this medication are the potential for abuse and difficulty with later withdrawal of the drug.

Obsessive-Compulsive Disorder

This disorder is more frequent than originally thought—surveys indicate that it affects 1%-2% of the population. The illness is characterized by either the presence of intrusive, repetitive, unwanted (and often distasteful) thoughts, or the presence of repetitive, excessive behaviors (e.g., washing, checking, counting) that the patient performs in a stereotyped or ritualized manner in order to prevent anxiety or an imagined dreaded outcome. Antidepressants with strong serotonergic effects are proving to be helpful in the treatment of this disorder. Clomipramine is the only drug that is approved by the Food and Drug Administration (FDA) for this purpose; however, fluoxetine may be equally effective. Fluvoxamine is not yet available in the United States, but also appears to be effective. Some patients do not respond to treatment with either clomipramine or fluoxetine; some clinicians have found that the addition of trazodone or buspirone may be effective for these patients. This should be done cautiously.

Posttraumatic Stress Disorder

This disorder may occur in people who have suffered a very traumatizing event. The symptoms include psychological reexperiencing of the trauma, avoidance of stimuli or situations that are associated with the trauma, and increased emotional or physiologic arousal.

Table 1–14.
Nonextrapyramidal CNS Side Effects of Neuroleptics*

Syndrome	Features	Period of Maximum Risk	Proposed Mechanism	Treatment	Common Offenders
Central anticholingeric syndrome	Toxic psychosis (delirium)	Weeks	Central anticholinergic excess	Stop or decrease anticholinergic, antiparkinsonian antidepressant, and antipsychotic agents	Thioridazine, chlorpromazine, low-potency agents others; caution in elderly and organically impaired
Neuroleptic malignant syndrome ("lethal catatonia")	Change in mental status; autonomic instability of vital signs in any combination (pulse, BP, temperature, respiration, ± diaphoresis); rigidity, increased creatine phosphokinase; myoglobinemia; lethal in 20% syndrome develops over 24–72 hr	Unpredictable can occur idio-idiosyncratically even after years of neuroleptic treatment	? Hypothalamic interference with temperature and vital signs regulation	Early detection; any 1 or more of the features listed (especially vital signs and mental status should alter staff; stop neuroleptic; antiparkinsonian agents usually fail;bromocriptine often helps dantrolene variable; parenteral benzodiazepines sometimes help; general supportivecare crucial (usually ICU setting)	All agents

Temperature dysregulation	Hyperthermia, hypothermia	Affected by environmental temperature extremes and activity level	? Peripheral interference with temperature regulation	Stop drug; rule out "lethal cataonia", cooling, techniques, massage; other supportive treatment for hyperthermia	All agents
Decrease in seizure threshold	Seizure activity is rare	Weeks	? Anticholinergic	Minimize dose; slowly increase if necessary; anticonvulsants	Chlorpromazine, promazine; low-potency agents > others, especially at high or rapidly rising dosage; molindone and piperazines least

*Adapted from Baldessarini RJ: *Chemotherapy in Psychiatry:* Cambridge, Mass, Harvard University Press, 1985; and Lydiard RB, et al in Gold MS, et al (eds): *Advances in Psychopharmacology*. Boca Raton, Fla, CRC Press, 1984.

Table 1–15.
General Guidelines to Treat Extrapyramidal Symptoms*†

Medication (po, mg)	Dose Range (mg/day)	Dosing Interval	Mechanism of Action	Common Side Effects
Benztropine mesylate (Cogentin), 1 and 2	1–8	BID–QID	Anticholin, antihistaminic	Dry mouth, blurred vision, impaired sweating,
Biperiden (Akineton), 2	2–10	TID–QID	Antichol	Constipation, memory and concentration impairment
Procyclidine hydrochloride (Kemadrin),5	5–20	TID–QID	Antichol	Urinary retention, tachycardia, anticholinergic delirium, contraindication with narrow-angle glaucoma
Trihexyphenidyl (Artane), 2 and 5	2–12	QID		
Diphenhydramine hydrochloride (Benadryl), 25 and 50	25–200	QID	Antichol, antihistaminic	Also sedation with diphenhydramine hydrochloride
Amantadine hydrochloride (Symmetrel), 100	200–300	BID–TID	Dopamine agonist	May exacerbate psychotic symptoms
Bromocriptine mesylate (Parlodel), 2.5 and 5.0	2.5–10	q.d.–BID	Dopamine agonist	Headache, constipation confusion, nausea
Clonazepam (Klonopin), 0.5, 1.0, 2.0	0.5–8.0	BID	Sedation? anxiolytic? GABA-ergic?	Sedation, ataxia

Lorazepam (Ativan), 0.5, 1.0, 2.0	1–10	TID–QID	Sedation? anxiolytic? GABA-ergic?	Sedation, ataxia
Propranolol hydrochloride (Inderal), 10, 20, 40, 60 and 80	20–120	QID	β-Blocker	Sedation, depression, bradycardia, hypotension
Reserpine (Serpasil), 0.1 and 0.25	0.1–1.0	q.d.–BID	Catecholamine depletion	Sedation, depression, bradycardia, hypotension
Baclofen (Lioresal), 10	15–60	TID	GABA?	Sedation
Methyldopa (Aldomet), 125, 250, and 500	250–2,000	QID	Block catecholamine synthesis	Sedation, depression, hypotension

* Adapted from Guze BH (ed): *The Handbook of Psychiatry*. Chicago, Year Book, 1990, p 422.
†Anticholin = anticholinergie; GABA = γ = aminobutyric acid.

There are no specific pharmacologic treatments for this disorder; however, selected patients with prominent symptoms of anxiety or depression may benefit from treatment with anxiolytics (buspirone or benzodiazepines) or antidepressants.

Phobic Disorders

These disorders are characterized by exaggerated and irrational fears. They are common; occurring in about 6% of the US population. Phobic disorders are divided into three categories: agoraphobia, social phobia, and simple phobias.

Agoraphobia is characterized by fear of situations from which escape might be difficult or help might not be available. Frequently, the patient will gradually and increasingly restrict his or her activities outside of the home. This disorder usually develops as a complication of panic disorder. Accordingly, agoraphobia is usually treated like panic disorder, i.e., treatment with antidepressants. Alprazolam, and possibly other benzodiazepines, may also be effective, though caution regarding abuse potential is warranted.

Social phobia is characterized by the persistent fear of being scrutinized by others, or of being humiliated or embarrassed. There is no specific treatment for this disorder, though there are a number of reports of successful treatment with antidepressants, especially MAOIs.

Simple phobias have also occasionally been treated with antidepressants (especially MAOIs); however, the efficacy of this treatment has not been established. Behavior modification therapy continues to be the mainstay of treatment for simple phobias.

Performance anxiety, associated with public speaking or performance, does not usually meet DSM-III-R* criteria for an anxiety disorder, but nevertheless can be an extremely troubling symptom. Low doses of β-blockers (e.g., propranolol), administered prior to the feared performance, are often helpful. However, this treatment has also not been well established in the scientific literature. Some clinicians have also found β-blockers to be helpful in other anxiety states in which symptoms of motor tension and autonomic arousal predominate.

*American Psychiatric Association: *Diagnostic and Statistical Manual of Mental Disorders DSM-III-R*, ed 3, rev. Washington, DC, American Psychiatric Association, 1987.

EATING DISORDERS

Anorexia Nervosa

This disorder is characterized by a refusal to maintain a body weight of at least 85% of expected normal weight, an intense fear of gaining weight or becoming fat, a disturbance in body image (e.g., perceiving oneself as fat in spite of being clearly underweight), and, in women, a loss of menstruation for at least three cycles. The primary treatments are refeeding programs followed by individual, group, and behavioral therapies. No clearly effective pharmacologic treatment has been found. Some research and case reports suggest that a modest weight gain can be achieved with cyproheptadine (a serotonin and histamine antagonist) at doses of about 32 mg/day, or with naltrexone (an opiate antagonist) with doses of 50 to 150 mg/day. Patients with associated depression have shown response to treatment with tricyclic antidepressants or fluoxetine. Pharmacologic treatment of patients with anorexia nervosa needs to be done cautiously since they may develop high drug blood levels more rapidly than usual, and they may be particularly sensitive to side effects (e.g., orthostatic hypotension).

Bulimia Nervosa

The symptoms of this disorder are recurrent episodes of binge eating, and regular but drastic attempts at weight control via laxatives, diuretics, self-induced vomiting, fasting, or vigorous exercise. Patients with this disorder have high frequencies of coexisting depression or anxiety disorder. Tricyclic antidepressants appear to be helpful in treatment even when coexisting affective illness is not present. Some clinicians feel that desipramine may be especially effective. Fluoxetine, lithium, and MAOIs also show some promise, though their effectiveness has not been established. Some nonantidepressants, including phenytoin, carbamazepine, and naltrexone, may also help to reduce bulimic behavior, but controlled studies are still needed.

SLEEP DISORDERS

DSM-III-R divides sleep disorders into two categories: dyssomnias and parasomnias. The former relate to disorders of the amount or timing of sleep, and can be subdivided into insomnias and hypersomnias; the latter relate to abnormal or pathologic events that occur as part of sleep. Pharmacologic interventions are rarely used for the parasomnias. Time, education, reassurance, and behavior modification are usually the first lines of treatment. Occasionally, tricyclic antidepressants are helpful in the treatment of chronic, refractory, childhood enuresis. There is some evidence that benzodiazepines may be helpful for severe night terrors.

Insomnia

Insomnia is the most common of sleep disorders; 10% to 15% of the US population describe insomnia as a major problem in their lives. Short-term insomnias of less than 1 months's duration can usually be helped by a combination of counseling, addressing stressful situations, and, if necessary, short-term use of hypnotic medications. Benzodiazepines (rather than other hypnotic drugs) are preferable for the treatment of insomnia (see Table 1–16). The benzodiazepine often is only necessary for a few days, but on occasion, continued use for 2 to 3 weeks may be indicated. When use for more than a few days is required, it is preferable to administer the drug intermittently, in order to avoid problems with tolerance and withdrawal insomnia.

Selection of a specific benzodiazepine is primarily determined by the length of action of the drug, though there may also be some variation in the sedative efficacy among the benzodiazepines. Longer-acting benzodiazepines, such as flurazepam and quazepam, may produce less withdrawal insomnia, but they have more problems with daytime sedation and poorer tolerance in the elderly (with slowed elimination, building blood levels, and subsequent confusion). Shorter-acting benzodiazepines, such as lorazepam, oxazepam, temazepam, and triazolam, are often better tolerated, but they may have greater problems with rebound or withdrawal insomnia. They may also be less effective with insomnia problems that occur toward the end of the night's sleep.

Long-term insomnias of greater than 3 to 4 week's duration require a thorough medical and psychiatric evaluation before instituting treatment. After organic causes and primary psychiatric disorders have been ruled out, treatment is focused on patient education regarding sleep hygiene and behavioral interventions. Hypnotic drugs are used as a short-term (less than 1 month) adjunct to these treatments, when it is necessary to help overcome a patient's high level of anticipatory anxiety regarding not falling asleep.

Table 1–16.
Benzodiazepines*

Generic Name	Primary Metabilic Pathway	Elimination Half-Life (hr)	Active Metabolites	Recommended Total Adult Daily Dose
Dizapepam	Oxidation	10–100	Diazepam, desmethyldiazepam	4–40 mg
Chlordiazepoxide	Oxidation	10–100	Chloridiazeproxide, desmethylchloridia- zepoxide, demoxepam, desmethyldiazepam	15–100 mg
Chlorazepate	Oxidation	30–100	Desmethyldiazepam	15–60 mg
Halazepam	Oxidation	15–100	Halazepam, desmethyldiazepam	60–120 mg
Prazepam	Oxidation	30–100	Desmethyldiazepam	20–60 mg
Alprazolam	Oxidation	10–16	Alprazolam	0.75–1.5 mg
Lorazepam	Conjugation	10–30	None	2–6 mg
Oxazepam	Conjugation	5–15	None	30–120 mg
Flurazepam	Oxidation	47–100	Hydroxyethylflurazepam, desalkylflurazepam, diazepam	15–30 mg

Table 1–17.
Dosing Information for Stimulants in Treatment of Attention-Deficit Hyperactivity Disorder*

Drug (Age Limit)	Starting Dose (mg/day)	Increment (mg/day)	Interval Between Increases	Maximum Dose (mg/day)	Average Dose (mg/day)	Average Dose (mg/kg/day)
Methylphennidate (Ritalin) (> 6 yr)	5–10	5–10	3–7 days	60–80	20–20	1.0–2.0
Dextroamphetamine (Dexedrine)						
(3–5 yr)	2.5	2.5	3–7 days			0.15–0.50
(≥ 6 yr)	2.5–1.0	5.0	3–7 days	40	10–20	0.15–0.50
Pemoline (Cylert)						
(>6 yr)	18.75–37.5	18.75	1 wk	112.5	50–75	0.5–2.0

*Adapted from Guze BH (ed): *The Handbook of Psychiatry*. Chicago, Year Book, 1990, p 411.

Hypersomnia

Hypersomnias are conditions of excessive daytime sleepiness. In some cases they may be caused by a condition that disturbs nighttime sleep, e.g., sleep apnea. Sedative medications administered during the night may worsen this condition. Generally, these patients require expert evaluation. Tricyclic antidepressants and medroxyprogesterone may be helpful in some patients (see Table 1–2). Some patients require surgical interventions or the administration of nighttime continuous positive airway pressure (CPAP).

Narcolepsy is a hypersomnia disorder. CNS stimulants such as methylphenidate, pemoline, and dextroamphetamine help to control the excessive sleepiness (Table 1–17). Tricyclic antidepressants, such as imipramine or protriptyline may help to control other, rapid eye movement (REM)–related symptoms: cataplexy, hypnagogic hallucinations, and sleep paralysis (Table 1–2).

ANTI-DEPRESSANTS 2

Tricyclic Antidepressants

GENERAL STATEMENT

History

During the 1950s there was extensive clinical testing of phenothiazine analogues. One of these analogues, imipramine, was discovered by R. Kuhn to be rather ineffective in the treatment of psychosis, but remarkably helpful in the treatment of depression.

Pharmacology

The precise mechanism of the antidepressant action of tricyclic antidepressants (TCAs) is unknown; however, it is known that these drugs block reuptake of various neurotransmitters, especially dopamine, serotonin, and norepinephrine, at the neural synapse. This action potentiates the effects of these biogenic amines. Furthermore, many TCAs exhibit strong anticholinergic effects. It has been suggested that the antidepressant effects may relate to any or all of these actions; however, most authorities believe that the effects on norepinephrine and serotonin are the principle ones. The reuptake blocking action of the TCAs is distinct from the actions of the monoamine oxidase inhibitors (MAOIs)—TCAs do not block oxidative deamination of the monoamines. Cyclic antidepressants may lower seizure threshold and result in an increased alpha activity and a decline in theta activity on the electroencephalogram (EEG). They also increase stage 4 sleep while markedly inhibiting rapid eye movement (REM) sleep. Some investigators believe the REM suppression may be crucial to the antidepressant action. Cyclic antidepressants may produce a variety of effects on other organ systems, especially the cardiovascular system. These effects include changes in cardiac conduction, tachycardia, and postural hypotension. These may result from their direct quinidine-like effects and from indirect cardiac effects secondary to anticholinergic activity and increased noradrenergic activity.

Pharmacokinetics

Absorption. TCAs are well absorbed from the gastrointestinal (GI) tract. There is, however, considerable individual variation in resulting plasma levels. This may be due to genetic differences in either the rate of drug metabolism or in differences in the amount of drug bound to plasma protein. The American Psychiatric Association has concluded that monitoring plasma concentrations of imipramine, nortriptyline, and desipramine is useful in patients who do not respond to the usual dosages, in patients at risk for development of toxicity either because of age or preexisting illness, in individuals in whom treatment is considered urgent, such as potentially suicidal patients, and in those patients whose illness may jeopardize their work or ability to care for their family. Blood levels may also be helpful in assessing compliance. There are, however, insufficient data at this point to recommend monitoring plasma concentrations for other TCAs.

Distribution. TCAs and their active metabolites are bound to plasma proteins and tissue proteins. They cross the placenta. Amitriptyline, amoxapine, desipramine, imipramine, nortriptyline, and doxepin are known to be distributed into breast milk; this probably holds true for other TCAs as well.

Elimination. TCAs are metabolized in the liver by N-demethylation, N-oxidation, aromatic and aliphatic hydroxylation, dealkylation, and conjugation. Some metabolites such as N-monodemethylated derivatives are lipophilic and can cross the blood-brain barrier. Because of this they are pharmacologically active. However, polar metabolites are pharmacologically less active; these are usually formed by oxidation or hydroxylation. Lipophilic metabolites are reabsorbed and remetabolized, whereas nonlipophilic metabolites are excreted in feces via the bile, or by urinary excretion.

Steady-state half-lives and rates of elimination vary widely among TCAs and among individuals. For example, the average half-life for amitriptyline is 16 hours, compared to 80 hours for protriptyline.

Uses

Depressive Disorders. TCAs are used to treat major depressive disorders. They may also be used to treat the depressive phase of bipolar affective disorder; however, they do not prevent and may precipitate manic or hypomanic attacks in bipolar patients. No one TCA has been demonstrated to have a decisive clinical superiority over another.

TCAs may be used in conjunction with electroconvulsive therapy (ECT). It has been reported that this may reduce the number of ECT treatments required. However, subjects may be at greater risk for the development of either hypomania or a toxic delirium. In most cases TCAs are considered the first line of treatment for major depression; other novel agents may be indicated in certain cases. MAOIs are generally reserved for those patients who have not benefited from TCAs or have an atypical depression. Concurrent use of a TCA and an MAOI is controversial; many authorities believe the combination should be avoided. However, when used in combination, it has been suggested that the MAOI therapy be started at least 2 days after TCAs have been initiated, and dosages of both agents should be increased gradually. In these cases parenteral administration should be avoided as should large quantities of either drug. The patient should be carefully monitored for side effects, including elevated blood pressure.

Other Psychiatric Disorders. TCAs may be of benefit in the treatment of psychotic depressions. In this case TCAs are used in conjunction with neuroleptic antipsychotic drugs. However, many clinicians feel that ECT is the treatment of choice for depressions with psychotic features.

TCAs are often used in conjunction with benzodiazepines in the treatment of anxious depressions. Tricyclic antidepressants are effective in the treatment of anxiety syndromes, including phobic and panic disorders. This action appears to be independent of their antidepressant efficacy. Tricyclics have also been suggested for the treatment of alcoholism and eating disorders (especially bulimia). In these cases it is less clear that the benefits are independent of the antidepressant action.

TCAs have been used in the treatment of attention deficit disorder with hyperactivity, but, they are generally considered to be inferior to methylphenidate in their clinical efficacy.

Imipramine hydrochloride has been used in the treatment of enuresis in children over the age of 6 years.

Clomipramine, a TCA recently approved by the Food and Drug Administration (FDA), is effective in the treatment of obsessive-compulsive disorder. Similar effectiveness is being found with other, new serotonergic antidepressants. Though not clearly established, the TCAs may also have important roles in the treatment of chronic pain, migraine, neuralgias, sleep apnea, narcolepsy, and peptic ulcer disease.

Cautions

Adverse Effects. Adverse effects of TCAs are usually mild, of short duration, and rarely require discontinuation of the antidepressant. In most cases tolerance develops to the anticholinergic, and postural hypotension effects. The incidence of adverse side effects can be minimized by initiating therapy at a low dose and gradually titrating upward.

Anticholinergic Effects. Anticholinergic effects are the most common adverse effect of TCAs. These include dry mouth, blurred vision, constipation, tachycardia, urinary retention, and difficulty initiating urination. The last is of special concern in men with prostatic hypertrophy. Anticholinergic effects are most common and most problematic in geriatric patients.

Nervous System Effects. Adverse central nervous system (CNS) effects are not uncommon. Drowsiness occurs frequently; weakness, lethargy, and fatigue may also occur. In some patients, however, there may be insomnia, restlessness, excitement, and agitation. In particular, in the geriatric population, impaired concentration, confusion, disorientation, delusions, and hallucinations may occur. Children seem to be at greatest risk for developing emotional lability, nervousness, sleep disorders, and either drowsiness or anxiety. Exacerbation of hypomania or panic may occur in patients receiving TCAs. Likewise, patients with bipolar disorder may shift to the manic phase. Alteration in EEGs have occurred and less commonly seizures develop. Extrapyramidal symptoms occur rarely; most commonly a fine tremor is seen in both young and old patients. A parkinsonian-like syndrome may occur in patients who are elderly and receiving high doses. Tardive dyskinesia has been associated with amoxapine therapy. Amoxapine has also been associated with neuroleptic malignant syndrome.

Cardiovascular Effects. Postural hypotension, the result of peripheral α-adrenergic blockade, is common during treatment with TCAs, especially in the elderly. Other cardiac effects stem from the quinidine-like effect of TCAs and include depression of the myocardium, prolonged conduction times, inversion or flattening of the T wave, and other abnormalities. Conduction disturbances are usually manifest as a bundle-branch block or atrioventricular (AV) block; therefore, these medications should only be used with special caution and with electrocardiographic (ECG) monitoring in patients who have these ECG abnormalities. In addition, patients may experience tachycardia or bradycardia, palpitations, and ventricular extrasystoles. In overdose, these cardiac effects can be potentially fatal.

Hematologic Effects. Agranulocytosis, thrombocytopenia, leukopenia, and eosinophilia have rarely been reported in patients receiving TCAs.

Hepatic Effects. Jaundice and hepatitis have been reported; they appear to be reversible upon discontinuation of the drug. Jaundice is of an obstructive type. The hepatitis appears to be allergic in nature. There is often an asymptomatic increase in transaminases and changes in alkaline phosphatase.

Sensitivity Reactions. Patients may develop photosensitivity and should either avoid exposure to sunlight or use a sunscreen. Some patients may manifest allergic reactions characterized by urticaria, pruritus, rash, and erythema. Sometimes these reactions are to the other compounds in the pills (e.g., dyes), rather than the actual drug.

Other Adverse Effects. Patients may manifest anorexia, nausea, vomiting, diarrhea, abdominal cramps, epigastric distress, and a peculiar taste in their mouth. Weight gain is a troublesome and frequent side effect; the mechanism is unclear. Both men and women may experience changes in libido; men may experience erectile impotence. Abrupt withdrawal of TCAs has been reported to precipitate a withdrawal syndrome characterized by anxiety, malaise, myalgias, chills, fever, nausea, vomiting, dizziness, headache, and possibly rebound dysphoria.

Precautions and Contraindications. TCAs may impair mental alertness or physical coordination. In light of this, patients should be cautioned about operating machinery, driving a motor vehicle, or engaging in other activities that require alertness or coordination. It should also be noted that TCAs exacerbate the effects of alcohol and possibly other sedatives.

TCAs are potentially lethal in overdose. Caution should be used in administering these drugs to suicidal patients or prescribing large amounts at one time.

TCAs lower the seizure threshold and should be used with caution in patients who have a history of seizure disorders.

Owing to the anticholinergic effects, subjects who could be harmed by anticholinergic activity should receive special consideration prior to the administration of TCAs. These are patients with benign prostatic hypertrophy, a history of urinary retention, or angle-closure glaucoma, for example.

Pregnancy, Fertility, and Lactation. There are no well-controlled studies on the effects of TCAs on the fetus. However, there have been some clinical reports of congenital malformation. The causal relationship in these cases is not clear. Nevertheless, when possible, these drugs should be avoided during pregnancy; ECT may be considered as a treatment alternative. It also appears that the TCAs are excreted in maternal milk; therefore, nursing women should not be treated with these drugs.

Overdosage and Toxicity

Pathogenesis. The average lethal dose for TCA in a young adult is approximately 30 mg/kg. In children this figure is 20 mg/kg. Children and patients with preexisting cardiovascular disease appear to be more susceptible to antidepressant-induced cardiotoxicity than healthy young adults.

Manifestations. Symptoms of overdose may occur anywhere from 1 to 2 hours after drug ingestion. Early features include hyperpyrexia, hallucinations, delirium, irritability, confusion, and agitation. Frequently there is myoclonus, choreiform movements, hypertension, hyperreflexia, nystagmus, and there may be a parkinsonian syndrome. As the overdose symptoms continue to progress, seizures may develop. Furthermore, urinary retention, dry mouth, mydriasis, flushed dry skin, and constipation with decreased bowel sounds may also develop as signs of peripheral anticholinergic overdose.

After an initial period of CNS stimulation, CNS depression may occur. During this period the patient may exhibit hyporeflexia or areflexia, drowsiness, hypothermia, hypotension, cyanosis, respiratory depression, and ultimately coma.

Cardiac rhythm abnormalities are common and may be life-threatening. These may include tachycardia and conduction disturbances. Cardiorespiratory arrest, congestive heart failure, and shock may also occur. In an overdose situation the quinidine-like effects may decrease intracardiac conduction. This decreased intraventricular conduction may be manifest by a prolonged QRS interval. A QRS interval longer than 100 ms may be the best indicator of severe overdose that may result in arrhythmias. However, it is possible to have a serious TCA overdose without evidence of substantial ECG abnormalities. Acidosis is the most frequent acid-base disturbance in tricyclic overdose. It may be metabolic, respiratory, or both in origin and usually results from hypotension, hypoventilation, or seizures.

Treatment. When patients have overdosed on a TCA they should be closely observed in a hospital setting—generally, an intensive care unit is best. Blood pressure should be monitored and there should be continuous ECG monitoring. Respiratory and cardiovascular function often require support, including endotracheal intubation. TCAs are usually removed from the GI tract by gastric lavage and the use of activated charcoal. Neither peritoneal dialysis nor hemodialysis are effective in removing TCAs because they are highly protein-bound. Seizures may be treated with benzodiazepines. Hypotension may be treated by elevating the feet and correcting the hypovolemia; the pressor effects of α-adrenergic agonists may be inhibited by the TCAs. Sodium bicarbonate may be given to maintain a normal systemic pH. Arrhythmias may be treated with lidocaine, phenytoin (also helps prevent seizures), or propranolol; quinidine procainamide and disopyramide should be avoided since these may further worsen cardiac conduction and contractility. There may be central and peripheral manifestations of anticholingeric excess. While these may make management more difficult, they are generally not life-threatening. Some clinicians have used physostigmine to reverse the anticholinergic symptoms including delirium; however, this is not considered safe in those more severe cases with instability of vital signs; and even in the milder cases its safety is controversial.

Drug Interactions

Monoamine Oxidase Inhibitors. Concomitant administration of TCAs and MAOIs may produce a hyperpyretic crisis, seizures, and death (Table 2–1). However, these have usually occurred in overdose situations or following parenteral administration. Following therapeutic dosages of these drugs given via oral administration, nonfatal hyperpyrexia, tachycardia, confusion, hypertension, and

Table 2–1.
Drug Interactions With Tricyclic Antidepressants (TCAs)

Combination	Interaction Effects	Mechanism/ Comments	Clinical Significance
Epinephrine and norepinephine (e.g., appetite suppressants, some local anesthetic formulations)	Enhanced cardiovascular effect into sympathetic neurons	TCAs inhibit epinephrine or norepinephrine reuptake	Yes
Alcohol	↑ Sedation and impairment of psychomotor skills and other TCA side effects	Synergistic effect (pronounced with more sedative drugs, e,g., amitriptyline)	Yes
	↓ TCA therapeutic effects	↑ Induction of microsomal enzyme (↑ metabolism of TCA)	Yes
	Impaired absorption of alcohol from gut	↓ Gastric emptying	
γ-Adrenergic agonist (norepinephrine)	↑ Pressor effect into sympathetic neurons	Potentiate action at peripheral receptor site	Yes
Amphetamines	↑ Stimulant effects	Potentiate at central receptor site	Yes
Analgestics (including antiinflammatory and antipyretic agents, e.g., phenazone, phenylbutazone)	↑ Phenazone action ↓ Phenylbutazone effect; ↑ risk of bone marrow depression	Inhibit phenazone metabolic enzyme, ↑ half-life ↓ gut motility → ↑ phenylbutazone absorption	Yes
Anesthetics (halothanes, pancuronium)	Tachyarrhythmias (case report: imipramine)	? Mechanism	?

(Continued.)

Table 2–1 (cont.)

Combination	Interaction Effects	Mechanism/ Comments	Clinical Significance
Anticholinergic drugs (e.g., antiemetic agents, antihistamines, atropine-like drugs, antiparkinsonian drugs)	↑ Anticholinergic effects/toxicity, esp. in geriatric patients (urinary retention, acute glaucoma, adynamic ileus)	Additive anticholingeric effects at receptor site	Yes
Anticoagulants (oral)	↑ Anticoagulant effect of coumarin drugs ↓ Anticoagulant and monitor protime	↓ Liver metabolism (↑ half-life)	Yes
Anticonvulsants	↑ Seizure risk	? Mechanism	?
Antihypertensives (e.g., guanethidine, bethanidine, debrisoquin, methyldopa, clonidine)	↑ Antihypersensitive effect, ↑ Dossage, or other hypotensive	Antagonism at receptor site; blood pressure drugs may not achieve satisfactory control except methyldopa	Yes
Antipsychotics	↑ Plasma TCA and antipsychotic (?) levels ↓ TCA toxicity	Possible inhibition of microsomal enzymes	?
Barbiturates bethanidine, debrisoquin,	↓ TCA therapeutic effects (↓ TCA plasma levels) May increase central and respiratory depressant effects	↑ Hepatic microsomal enzyme induction Shift to benzodiazepine or separate dosage of 2 drugs	?

(Continued.)

Baclofen	↑ Muscle weakness Avoid this combination	Imipramine and nortriptyline potentiate antispastic effect of baclofen	Yes
Benzodiazepines	↓ Side effects in low-dose combination	? Mechanism ↑ Sedation or atropine-like effects (TCA + chlordiazepoxide)	?
β-adrenergic agonists (epinephrine)	↑ Pressor effect	Additive at receptor site	Yes
β-adrenergic blockers	↓ Antihypertensive effects	↑ Antagonistic at receptor site	?
Carbamazepine	↓ Plasma TCA levels	↑ Metabolism	?
Chloramphenical	↑ Plasma TCA levels	↓ Metabolism	?
Cigarette smoking	↓ Plasma TCA levels	Hepatic microsomal induction	?
Cimetidine (histamine H_2 receptor antagonists)	↑ Plasma TCA levels and toxicity	↓ Hepatic clearance and ↑ bioavailability (inhibit both demethylation and hydroxylation) Ranitidine alternative to cimetidine ↓ TCA doses, if combination is necessary	Yes
CNS depressants	↑ Depressant effect	Potentiate at central receptor site	Yes
Cocaine (desipramine, imipramine, trazodone)	↓ Cocaine craving; desipramine blocks cocaine-induced euphoria	? Mechanism	?

(Continued.)

Table 2–1 (cont.).

Combination	Interaction Effects	Mechanism/ Comments	Clinical Significance
Disulfiram	↑ Plasma TCA levels Acute organic brain syndrome	↓ ? Metabolism 2 cases reported: amitriptyline	?
Enflurance	? ↑ Seizure risk	? Mechanism 2 cases reported: amitriptyline and enflurane	?
Estrogen	May augment TCA (imipramine) effects, both beneficial and adverse	Inhibits TCA metabolism ↓ Imipramine dose, or ↓ estrogen dose if TCA adverse effects are noted	?
Ethchlorvynol	Transient delirium	? Mechanism Cases reported	?
Fluoxetine	May increase pharmacologic and toxic effect of TCA	? Inhibition of TCA metabolism Symptoms and ↑ TCA levels may persist for several weeks after stoping fluoxetine	Yes
Griseofulvin	↓ Plasma TCA levels	↑ Metabolism	?
Levodopa	↑ Levodopa antiparkinsonian effects ↓ Gastric motility TCA impairs levodopa absorption in GI tract	Potentiate anticholinergic effects Imipramine and amitriptyline are safer for patient on levodopa	?

Lithium	↑ TCA antidepression effects If an interaction is suspected, taper or discontinue TCA and measure lithium blood levels	? Additive or synergistic effects	?
L-Triiodothyronine (T_3)	Accelerate or potentiate TCA effects ↑ Adverse effects of either agent	? Potentiate at central receptor site	?
MAOIs	Enhance clinical effect, toxicity Flushing, sweating, excitability, muscle twitchintg, tremor rigidity, opisthotonos; clonic and tonic convulsions, hyperpyrexia, headache, tachycardia, confusion, coma, disseminated intravascular coagulation, death	May be MAOI-induced block of enzymes which metabolize TCAs If both drugs are started simultaneously, add MAOI to TCA regimen and lower both doses; oral only; *imipramine, desipramine, and clomipramine should be avoided*	Yes
Methylphenidate (Ritalin)	↑ Plasma TCA level ↑ Clinical effects and toxicity	Inhibition of TCA metabolism or ? additive effects	Yes
Methyltestosterone (Metandren)	Paranoid ideation	? Mechanism 5 cases (men only) reported	Yes
Oral contraceptives	↓ Plasma TCA levels (↑ ?)	Hepatic microsomal induction (↓ metabolism?)	?

(Continued.)

Table 2–1 (cont.).

Combination	Interaction Effects	Mechanism/ Comments	Clinical Significance
Pethidine (meperidine), other narcotic analgesics	↑ Pethidine-induced respiratory depression	Similar interaction might be anticipated with all narcotic analgesics and other CNS depressants	Yes
Propoxyphene (Darvon), doxepin	↑ PlasmaTCA levels	Inhibition of oxidative metabolism Case report and animal study	?
Quinidine/quinine (Darvon)	↑ Certain TCA clinical effects and toxicity? Prolongation of cardiac conduction	Inhibit hepatic hydroxylation of certain TCAs Potentiate antiarrhythmic effects	?
Reserpine, rauwolfia alkaloids	↓ Reserpine hypotensive effect ↑ TCA initial improvement (?) Worsening of depression? (long-term effect)	Antagonism at receptor site Manic reaction reported	Yes
Sympathomimetic agents (amines)	↑ Pressor effects	Inhibition of norepinephrine reuptake Avoid concurrent use of sympathomimetic amines or (?) use of local anesthetic containing epinephrine or norepinephrine	Yes
Sulfonylureas	↑ Hypoglycemic reaction	? Mechanism Case report	?

seizures have been reported. Therefore, this combination should be used with caution and only in treatment-refractory cases. It is not clear that the combination is more efficacious than either drug alone.

CNS Agents. TCAs may potentiate the CNS depressant effects of alcohol, sedatives, or hypnotics. Barbiturates and nicotine may induce microsomal enzymes and increase hepatic metabolism of antidepressants. Thyroxine has been reported to accelerate the onset of therapeutic effects of TCAs. Methylphenidate may inhibit the metabolism of TCAs and increase their effectiveness. It is important to monitor anticholinergic effects when also using neuroleptics or antiparkinsonian drugs.

Other. The effects of toxicity of TCAs may be increased by drugs which competitively bind to plasma albumin: phenytoin, phenylbutazone, aspirin, phenothiazines, scopolamine, and aminopyrine. Other drugs can have similar effects by inhibiting hepatic breakdown including neuroleptics, oral contraceptives, and other steroids. TCAs may also inhibit the activity of the antihypertensives guanethidine and clonidine.

Drug interactions can affect the pharmacokinetics of a given drug at several different levels: absorption, distribution in body tissue, protein binding, metabolism, and excretion (pharmacokinetic interactions). Alterations in these parameters affect the levels of the drug at the action site and the action duration of the drug. In addition, drug interactions can occur at the receptor site, centrally or peripherally (pharmacologic or pharmacodynamic interaction), and result in one of four effects: additive (potentiated), synergistic, antagonistic, or no effect. Another form of drug interaction is idiosyncratic; it may lead to either a diminished therapeutic response of one of the drugs or the occurrence of a toxic or adverse effect of one drug in the combination. An allergic reaction is an example of this kind of drug interaction.

Several factors point to drug interactions as a paramount issue in psychopharmacology. The first is simply the burgeoning number of cases of clinically significant interactions. Further, in the last decade, the use of psychiatric medications by both psychiatrist and nonpsychiatric primary care physicians has increased, thus leading to a higher frequency of drug combinations and potential interactions. An additional factor is the growing number of geriatric patients, a high-risk group for significant drug interactions.

They are more sensitive to the adverse effects of any medication and many elderly patients are often prescribed multiple medications.

Heterocyclic antidepressants (especially TCAs) are often used in combination with other nonpsychiatric medications, and they are also probably the most common psychiatric agents prescribed for the elderly. There are increasing data documenting significant drug interactions with TCAs. These interactions can modify the pharmacologic action or pharmacokinetics of either the TCAs, the combined drugs, or both, thus causing a significant change in TCA blood levels, enhancing or diminishing the therapeutic effects or increasing the risk of unwanted or toxic effects.

Drug interactions for the major groups of antidepressants (TCAs and MAOIs) are listed in Tables 1–1 and 1–4. Comments are provided on the possible adverse effects, the underlying mechanisms, and the clinical significance. The following discussion provides additional clarification.

Tricyclic and Heterocyclic Antidepressants

Anticholinergic Agents. All of the currently marketed tricyclic and heterocyclic antidepressants possess considerable anticholinergic action, in particular, amitriptyline, doxepin, imipramine, maprotiline, nortriptyline, and trimipramine. Anticholinergic properties of heterocyclic antidepressants may potentiate both the central and peripheral effects of other agents with anticholinergic actions, such as antihistamines, antiparkinsonian drugs, atropine-like medications, glutethimide, meperidine (Demerol), and the phenothiazines. Combined use of heterocyclic antidepressants and other anticholinergics is not uncommon, at least in the elderly. Mental confusion may be the predominant symptom of excessive anticholinergic activity. The elderly are more vulnerable to anticholinergic effects, and, the possibility of precipitating acute glaucoma, adynamic ileus, or urinary retention should be considered. The physostigmine test is a useful diagnostic tool to assess anticholinergic toxicity due to antidepressant drugs.

CNS Depressants. Heterocyclic antidepressants (amitriptyline, doxepin, maprotiline, and trazodone in particular) may potentiate the CNS depressant effects of alcohol, barbiturates, benzodiazepines, and phenothiazines, producing excessive drowsiness and sedation. Several reports suggest that barbiturates decrease plasma levels of antidepressants. A large multicenter study showed a reduced frequency of complaints about side effects with the combined use of chlordiazepoxide and amitriptyline compared with either drug alone. However, the concurrent use of a benzodiazepine can increase the lethal effect of amitriptyline overdose without increasing plasma levels. With concomitant administration of TCAs and phenothiazines, the plasma level of TCAs may increase by up to 70%, with an increasing incidence of side effects, particularly in elderly patients. The most dangerous combination is TCA with thioridazine, both because of its potentiation of anticholinergic effects and its cardiac toxicity.

Cardiovascular Drugs. TCAs interact with anticoagulants, antihypertensive agents, antiarrhythmic drugs, and directly and indirectly acting pressor amines. By blocking the reuptake of norepinephrine at the presynaptic neuron, TCAs potentiate the hypertensive effects of both directly and indirectly acting pressor amines. Consequently, hypertensive crises, characterized by hyperthermia, sweating, severe headache, cerebrovascular accident, and death, have occurred from this interaction (see Table 2-/-1). TCAs antagonize the hypotensive effects of antihypertensive drugs such as methyldopa, clonidine, guanethidine, and reserpine, but rapid withdrawal of a TCA from a patient stabilized with these compounds can result in a serious hypotensive reaction. Hence, hypertension should be controlled before the commencement of a TCA, if possible by the use of diuretics or β-blockers, or both. The membrane-stabilizing effects of TCAs may be additive with a variety of antiarrhythmic drugs including quinidine, procainamide, and disopyramide. This additive interaction may cause depression of myocardial contractibility and congestive heart failure. Additionally, the quinidine-like agents may impair metabolism of the TCAs leading to toxicity. TCAs commonly induce postural hypotension, most likely due to relaxation of vascular smooth muscle, resulting in peripheral vasodilation. This hypotensive effect may be additive with a variety of vasodilator and antihypertensive agents, giving rising to uncomfortable and occasionally even dangerous hypotensive reactions.

Monoamine Oxidase Inhibitors. Concomitant administration of TCAs and MAOIs may produce a hyperpyretic crisis, seizure, and death. However, these have usually occurred in overdose situations or following parenteral administration. Following therapeutic dosage of these drugs given via oral administration, nonfatal hyperpyrexia, tachycardia, confusion, hypertension, and seizures have been reported. Although hypertensive reactions have been attributed to the interaction of MAOIs and TCAs, the risk of potentiated hypotension occurring with this combination is probably greater than the risk of a hypertensive reaction.

Miscellaneous. Anticonvulsant drugs, including phenobarbital and phenytoin, may increase the TCA metabolic rate, thereby decreasing the antidepressant effect. Stimulants such as amphetamines and methylphenidate inhibit TCA metabolism, consequently increasing both the serum level and the therapeutic response. Cimetidine inhibits hepatic metabolism of TCAs; it may increase the plasma levels of and therefore the risk of adverse effects and toxicity of the drug. Although the mechanism is uncertain, concurrent use of TCAs and levodopa may produce agitation, tremor and rigidity. L-Triiodothyronine has been reported to accelerate the onset of therapeutic effects of TCAs. Stimulants may inhibit the metabolism of TCAs, thereby increasing both the serum concentration and therapeutic response. Methylphenidate may inhibit the metabolism of TCAs and increase their effectiveness.

Dosage and Administration

Dosage. Dosage must be titrated to the individual's need, response, and side effects. There is a wide range of variation in TCA dosage requirements among individuals. Initially patients receive low doses of antidepressant; this is gradually increased upward as tolerated and needed. Therapeutic response may not occur until greater than 3 weeks beyond reaching a therapeutic dose of the drug. Duration of antidepressant treatment depends on the individual and his or her condition, but, it is not uncommon to continue antidepressant treatment 6 months beyond the initial remission of symptoms. It is controversial whether the antidepressant dosage should be reduced during this maintenance period. Recent studies indicate that relapse rates are lower if the initial, effective therapeutic dosage is continued throughout this period. To avoid withdrawal symptoms, termination of antidepressant medication should be effected as a gradual reduction in the daily dose administered. Ideally, we recommend a gradual reduction over a 1-month period.

Administration. TCAs are generally administered orally. Both imipramine hydrochloride and amitriptyline hydrochloride may also be given intramuscularly (IM). However, unless the patient is unable or unwilling to take the drug, IM administration offers no significant clinical advantage over oral administration. TCAs are long-acting. Because of this the entire dose may be given at one time, most commonly at bedtime. This may result in improved patient compliance. Administration of the entire dose at bedtime may promote sleep, minimize daytime sedation, and minimize difficulty with other side effects. In those patients who experience insomnia or general stimulation from TCAs, the entire dose may be given in the morning. In some cases, split dosing may help manage side effects.

AMITRIPTYLINE HYDROCHLORIDE

Pharmacokinetics

Absorption. Amitriptyline hydrochloride is rapidly absorbed from both parenteral injection sites and the GI tract with peak plasma concentrations being reached approximately 2 to 12 hours after oral or IM administration.

Distribution. Amitriptyline and its primary active metabolite nortriptyline are widely distributed, including into breast milk.

Elimination. The elimination half-life of amitriptyline can range from 10 to 50 hours. Metabolism occurs as discussed at the beginning of this chapter. Nortriptyline is an N-monodemethylated metabolite which is pharmacologically active. The administered amitriptyline is excreted in the urine as inactive metabolites. Within 24 hours approximately 25% to 50% of the administered dose undergoes this process.

Cautions

See under General Statement at the beginning of this chapter.

Dosage and Administration

Dosage. There is a wide individual variation in oral amitriptyline hydrochloride dosage requirements. Dosage must be individually titrated to the patient's specific need, tolerance, and side effects. Initial dosages for young adults usually are 50 to 100 mg/day depending on the patient's general physical condition and the severity of the condition being treated. In geriatric and adolescent patients the initial dose is usually 20 to 50 mg/day. Geriatric patients may do better with medications that have less anticholinergic and hypotensive effect.

Dosage is gradually adjusted upward to maximum therapeutic effect and may range as high as 300 mg/day. Antidepressant response may not occur until at least 3 weeks after initiation of drug treatment.

After resolution of depressive symptoms medication is titrated down to the lowest effective dosage. Maintenance therapy may persist as long as 6 months after the initial depressive episode. Care must be exercised in discontinuing an antidepressant in order to avoid symptoms of withdrawal. For this reason antidepressants should be discontinued gradually.

Amitriptyline is available in conjunction with phenothiazines in fixed-ratio combinations. These should be avoided during initial treatment. The dosage, instead, should be titrated individually for each drug. If, after this process is completed and the patient is stabilized, it is determined that the optimum maintenance dosage corresponds to the ratio available in the commercial compound, such a preparation may be used. However, if in the future additional adjustments in medication are necessary, each drug should be administered individually.

The usual IM dosage for amitriptyline hydrochloride in adults is 20 to 30 mg four times a day.

Administration. Amitriptyline hydrochloride is most commonly administered orally. Given its long-acting nature, the entire daily dose may be administered at one time. In addition, amitriptyline may be given parenterally as an IM injection. This should only be done in patients who are unwilling or unable to take amitriptyline orally. As soon as possible IM administration should be replaced by oral therapy.

Preparations

Amitriptyline hydrochloride

- Oral tablets (*Elavil, Endep*)
  - 10 mg, 25 mg, 50 mg, 75 mg, 100 mg, 150 mg
- Parenteral injection (*Elavil*)
  - 10 mg/mL chlordiazepoxide and amitriptyline hydrochloride (*Enovil*)

5 mg chlordiazepoxide and 12.5 mg amitriptyline hydrochloride (*Limbitrol*)
10 mg chlordiazepoxide and 25 mg
amitriptyline hydrochloride (*Limbitrol DS:* perphenazine and amitriptyline hydrochloride)

Oral tablets

2 mg perphenazine and 10 mg amitriptyline hydrochloride (*Triavil 2-10, Etrafon 2-10*)
2 mg perphenazine and 25 mg amitriptyline hydrochloride (*Triavil 2-25, Etrafon*)
4 mg perphenazine and 10 mg amitriptyline hydrochloride (*Triavil 4-10, Etrafon A*)
4 mg perphenazine and 25 mg amitriptyline hydrochloride (*Triavil 4-25*)
4 mg perphenazine and 50 mg amitriptyline hydrochloride (*Triavil 4-50, Etrafon Forte*)

AMOXAPINE

Pharmacokinetics

Absorption. Amoxapine is rapidly absorbed from the GI tract with peak plasma concentrations occurring at approximately 90 minutes after oral administration.

Distribution. Amoxapine is widely distributed through body tissues and is detected in human breast milk.

Elimination. The plasma half-life of amoxapine is approximately 8 hours. It is rapidly metabolized in the liver to 8-hydroxyamoxapine and to 7-hydroxyamoxapine. Both metabolites are pharmacologically active, the former having a half-life of 30 hours.

Uses

Amoxapine is used in the treatment of major depressions with and without symptoms of anxiety. Amoxapine appears to be equally effective with other TCAs. There have been some reports of amoxapine having a more rapid rate of onset. This, however, remains to be fully established.

Cautions

The usual precautions associated with TCA administration should be observed; these are reviewed in the General Statement above. Also of note is that extrapyramidal reactions have occurred in approximately 1% of patients receiving amoxapine. In addition, rarely, tardive dyskinesia has been reported in patients receiving the drug. Like other antipsychotic agents it may produce neuroleptic malignant syndrome (NMS). See the General Statement under neuroleptics regarding NMS.

Dosage and Administration

Dosage. Dosage must be titrated to the individual's need and tolerance. The usual effective dose is 200 to 300 mg/day. This is usually begun at 100 to 150 mg/day and titrated upward as tolerated. This is usually done during the first week of therapy. If there has been no significant improvement in depression and the patient has been taking the drug for 2 weeks at 300 mg/day, dosage may be increased up to a maximum of 400 mg/day in outpatients and, generally, up to 600 mg in inpatients, in those who do not have a history of seizures. Any single dose should not exceed 300 mg. Geriatric patients usually need lower average daily doses. In this population dosage should be initiated at 50 to 75 mg/day and increased to 100 to 150 mg/day by the end of the first week of therapy, if tolerated.

Antidepressant effects of amoxapine are usually noted after 2 to 3 weeks from initiation of drug treatment.

Administration. Amoxapine is administered orally. Due to its long half-life the entire daily dose may be administered once a day unless dosage exceeds 300 mg/day, in which case it should be given in divided doses.

Preparations

Amoxapine (*Asendin*)
  Oral tablets
    25 mg, 50 mg, 100 mg, 150 mg

BUPROPRION HYDROCHLORIDE

Buproprion is structurally distinct from the previously discussed antidepressants. It belongs to the aminoketone class. This unique chemical group is unrelated to tricyclic, tetracyclic, or other known antidepressants. It lacks both the polycyclic rings of most antidepressants and the functional groups common to most neuroleptics. Its chemical structure resembles that of diethylpropion. This is a sympathomimetic anorectic agent with stimulating properties. The neurochemical mechanism of action for the antidepressant effects of buproprion is unknown. It is a weak blocker of both norepinephrine and serotonin. It is not known to inhibit MAOIs. It has weak capabilities to inhibit the reuptake of dopamine into the neuron.

Pharmacokinetics

Absorption. Peak plasma concentrations are usually reached within 2 hours of drug administration. Only a small portion of the early administered dose reaches the circulation unmetabolized. This has been estimated to range in animals from 5% to 20% of the administered dose.

Distribution. In vitro tests show that buproprion is 80% or more bound to albumin. It appears to be widely distributed throughout the body.

Elimination. Drug elimination follows a biphasic decline. The average half-life of the second phase (postdistributional) is approximately 14 hours. Buproprion has pharmacologically active metabolites. At least two of these have longer elimination half-lives than the parent compound. Buproprion may induce its own metabolism. The steady-state concentrations of these metabolites are anywhere from 10 to 100 times the steady-state concentration of the parent drug. Buproprion is metabolized in the liver and excreted in the urine and feces. The elimination of the drug's metabolites may be affected by reduced hepatic function.

Uses

Buproprion is indicated for the treatment of depression. Its efficacy has not been established in systematic controlled trials for treatment longer than 6 weeks. During prolonged administration the physician should periodically examine the patient both for continued indication for drug treatment and to evaluate potential side effects. Evidence has begun to accumulate which suggests that buproprion may be helpful in bipolar illness. It may prevent a depressive recurrence and decrease the number of mood swing episodes. In other words there may be no increased cycling in bipolar patients. Buproprion may also be of some benefit in attention deficit disorder. However, it does not appear to be effective in the treatment of panic and agoraphobia.

Cautions

Adverse Effects. Patients not uncommonly complain of agitation, anxiety, restlessness, and insomnia as side effects from buproprion. These most commonly occur in the first few weeks after initiation of drug treatment. In a small percentage of patients (2%) these side effects may be severe enough to result in discontinuation of the drug. Other antidepressants are known to exacerbate bipolar disorder and psychosis. It is possible that buproprion may in some patients produce delusions, hallucinations, or other psychotic symptoms and may in theory activate mania. Approximately 28% of patients taking buproprion will experience a weight loss greater than 5 lb. In contrast, approximately 9.4% of patients will experience a weight gain; this compares to approximately 34.5% of patients who gain weight while receiving a TCA. The weight loss potential may be significant in patients who have already experienced significant weight loss as a symptom of their depressive disease.

Buproprion should be used with caution in patients who have significant renal or hepatic impairment. In these patients the medication should be started at reduced initial dosage and the patient should be closely monitored for the development of side effects. The use of buproprion in patients with a recent history of unstable heart disease or myocardial infarction has not been established. Care should be used if the drug is administered to these patients.

The risk of *seizures* in patients treated with buproprion is approximately 0.4% in patients treated at doses up to 450 mg/day. This is greater than the risk found with other antidepressants by as much as four times. The risk of seizure occurrence increases approximately tenfold as doses increase between 450 and 600 mg/day. Doses in this range should be used with caution. The risk of seizure development is associated with both dose and the presence of predisposing factors. Predisposing factors include a history of head trauma or prior seizures, concomitant medications that lower the seizure threshold, CNS tumor, or other CNS lesions. These have been present in approximately half of the patients experiencing a seizure. An additional risk may be a rapid or large increase in dosage. Seizures may occur at any time during the course of treatment, but most commonly they occur during the early course of treatment. The risk of seizure may be minimized by several factors. The daily dose of buproprion should not exceed 450 mg/day. Furthermore, this dose should be administered three times a day with each single dose not to exceed 150 mg. This is done to avoid high serum concentrations of buproprion or its metabolites. Increases in dosage should be performed gradually. Bulimia appears to be an additional risk factor for the development of seizures. Not as well established, but probably also significant is anorexia nervosa. For this reason buproprion should not be administered to patients either with bulimia nervosa or anorexia nervosa.

Pregnancy, Fertility, Lactation. Buproprion is distributed into breast milk. Because of this a decision should be made whether to discontinue the medication or discontinue nursing in breast-feeding patients receiving buproprion.

Animal studies using up to 45 times the human dose have failed to reveal definite impairment of either fertility or fetal harm associated with buproprion. These drugs should be used in pregnant women only if the therapeutic benefit clearly exceeds the risk.

Toxicity

Side effects commonly associated with the administration of buproprion include insomnia, nausea, vomiting, headache (including migraines), constipation, tremor, and dry mouth. Approximately 10% of patients may find side effects sufficiently problematic that they elect to discontinue the drug. These adverse reactions are more likely to occur with higher doses of the drug, in particular in doses that exceed the recommended daily dose. Other frequent side effects occurring in approximately 1% of patients include edema, nonspecific rashes, nocturia, ataxia and incoordination, seizures, myoclonus, dyskinesia, and dystonia. There may be flu-like symptoms, stomatitis, mania or hypomania, increased libido, hallucinations, decrease in sexual function, and depression.

There have been a limited number of overdoses associated with buproprion. In patients ingesting large quantities of buproprion alone (up to 4,200 mg) there has been recovery without significant sequelae. However, in higher doses (9,000 mg), and in those associated with tranylcypromine there have been grand mal seizures and, likewise, recovery without further sequelae. Patients suspected of overdose should be hospitalized. Gastric lavage is indicated; induction of emesis is best avoided because of the risk of aspiration. Activated charcoal may help in the first 12 hours after ingestion. Baseline ECGs and EEGs are recommended with serial monitoring during the next 48 hours. Adequate hydration should be insured. If the patient is stuporous, comatose, or convulsing, then gastric lavage along with airway intubation is recommended. Lavage is likely to be of benefit during the first 12 hours after ingestion.

Dosage and Administration

Dosage. The usual adult dosage is 300 mg/day divided into three doses. Dosing should begin at 200 mg/day, given as 100 mg twice a day. This may be titrated upward to 300 mg/day administered as 100 mg three times a day if clinically indicated. This should be done no sooner than 3 days after beginning therapy. The full antidepressant effect of buproprion may not be observed until 4 weeks after initiation of drug treatment. If, after several weeks of treatment at 300 mg/day, there has been no clinical improvement, then consideration can be given to increasing the dose up to a maximum of 450 mg/day given in divided doses of not more than 150 mg each. The 100-mg tablet may be administered four times a day with at least 4 hours between successive doses. Or multiples of the 75-mg tablets may be used to achieve 450 mg/day. Buproprion should be discontinued in patients who do not demonstrate an adequate therapeutic response after an extended period of treatment at 450 mg/day. Lower doses should be used in the elderly and in adolescents. The safety and effectiveness of buproprion has not been established for patients 18 years or age or younger, however.

Administration. Buproprion is administered orally. Increases in dosage should not exceed 100 mg/day in a 3-day period. Gradual escalation in dosage is important if agitation, restlessness, and insomnia are seen during the initial days of treatment. Gradual increases in dosage will minimize the side effects. These side effects may be further managed by either a temporary reduction of the administered dose of buproprion or by the coadministration of a long-acting sedative-hypnotic. Likewise, administration of buproprion in the morning will minimize insomnia. No single dose of buproprion should exceed 150 mg; doses of this size should be separated by at least 6 hours.

Preparations

Buproprion hydrochloride (*Wellbutrin*)
Oral tablets
75 mg, 100 mg

CLOMIPRAMINE HYDROCHLORIDE

In the United States, clomipramine is used primarily as an antiobsessional drug. Clomipramine is believed to exert its antiobsessional effects through a modification of serotonergic synaptic transmission.

Pharmacokinetics

Absorption. Peak plasma levels of clomipramine occur approximately 4.7 hours after drug administration.

Distribution. Clomipramine is distributed widely throughout the body. It is found in cerebrospinal fluid (CSF) and breast milk. It is approximately 97% protein-bound. The interaction between clomipramine and other highly protein-bound drugs may be clinically important.

Elimination. Clomipramine is metabolized to desmethylclomipramine, which is an active metabolite. The effects of desmethylclomipramine on obsessive-compulsive behaviors is unknown. Following biliary elimination metabolites are excreted in the feces and in urine. The elimination half-lives of clomipramine and desmethylclomipramine may considerably lengthen at doses near the upper end of the recommended dosing range (i.e., 200–250 mg/day), potentially causing clomipramine and desmethylclomipramine to accumulate. This may increase the incidence of dose-dependent adverse reactions. The mean elimination half-lives of clomipramine and desmethylclomipramine are 32 and 69 hours, respectively. Steady-state levels are achieved within 7 to 14 days for clomipramine. The effects of hepatic and renal impairment on the elimination of clomipramine have yet to be determined.

Uses

Clomipramine is indicated for the treatment of severe obsessive-compulsive disorder. The obsessions or compulsions should significantly interfere with social or occupational functioning, be time-consuming, or cause marked distress. Obsessions are recurrent persistent thoughts, ideas, images, or impulses that are ego-dystonic. Compulsions are repetitive, intentional, purposeful behaviors performed in response to an obsession in a stereotyped fashion and are recognized by the patient as excessive or unreasonable. The effectiveness of clomipramine in trials greater than 10 weeks' duration has not been evaluated in systematic placebo-controlled trials. Patients treated for extended periods should be periodically reevaluated for the usefulness of continued treatment.

Cautions

The manufacturer recommends that clomipramine hydrochloride not be administered within 14 days of treatment with an MAOI. The manufacturer states that hyperpyretic crisis, seizures, coma, and death have been reported in patients receiving such combinations.

Clomipramine is contraindicated in patients during the acute recovery period after a myocardial infarction.

During premarketing evaluation the cumulative incidence of seizures increased with continued exposure to clomipramine. In doses up to 300 mg/day the seizure risk was 0.64% at 90 days, 1.12% at 180 days, and 1.45% at 365 days. Both dose and duration of exposure appear to be significant risks for predicting a seizure. The manufacturer recommends a maximum dose of 250 mg in adults and 3 mg/kg (or 200 mg) in children and adolescents to minimize the risk of seizure. Clomipramine should be used with extreme caution in patients with a history of seizure disorders, and in those with such predisposing factors as brain damage, alcoholism, or concomitant use of other drugs that lower the seizure threshold.

Patients should be cautioned about engaging in hazardous activity including operating machinery or driving an automobile where sedation or sudden loss of consciousness could result in serious injury to the patient or others.

Changes in the ECG are uncommon. When they occur the most common findings are the development of premature ventricular contractions (PVCs), ST-T wave changes, and intraventricular conduction abnormalities. These changes are usually clinically asymptomatic. Caution should be used, however, in patients with known cardiovascular disease.

Clomipramine may induce hypomania or mania. Rarely, clomipramine is associated with significant elevations in aspartate (AST, SGOT) and alanine (ALT, SGPT) aminotransferases. At times these may exceed three times the upper limit of normal. In most cases the increased levels are not associated with significant clinical findings. There have, however, been reports of severe liver injury associated with clomipramine administration. Weight gain occurs in approximately 18% to 20% of patients taking clomipramine. Approximately 25% of these patients will gain greater than 7% of their initial body weight. Approximately 5% of patients will lose at least 7% of their initial body weight.

Sexual dysfunction in male patients treated with clomipramine is frequent. Forty-two percent of patients experienced ejaculatory failure and 20% experienced erectile impotence during premarketing evaluation.

Toxicity

Toxic manifestations are similar to other TCA, with the most common, problems being dry mouth, constipation, nausea, somnolence, tremor, nervousness, myoclonus, impotence, impaired urination, fatigue, sweating, alterations in appetite, weight gain, and blurred vision.

Overdosage. The development of signs and symptoms in the overdose situation are dependent on dose, age of the patient, and the time since drug ingestion. Early signs are usually severe anticholinergic reactions. Abnormalities may include drowsiness, stupor, coma, ataxia, restlessness, agitation, delirium, and hyperactive reflexes that may progress to myoclonus and convulsions. Cardiac abnormalities may include arrhythmias, tachycardias, and ECG evidence of delayed cardiac conduction. Treatment should consist of maintenance of adequate respiration and circulation, accompanied by close observation, including continuous cardiac monitoring. Physostigmine may be of benefit in reversing the cardiovascular and anticholinergic manifestations of overdosage. However, it may induce seizures and a cholinergic crisis. Efforts should be made to prevent further gut absorption of the drug by gastric lavage and use of activated charcoal. Induction of emesis is generally not recommended because of the risk of aspiration. Administration of anticonvulsants may also be necessary.

Drug Interactions

There is little systematic information regarding the use of clomipramine with other drugs. In general, caution should be used with the MAOIs. Concomitant administration with haloperidol may elevate the plasma concentration of clomipramine. Methylphenidate, fluoxetine, and cimetidine may also raise the serum level of clomipramine. Caution should be used in the administration of drugs which are highly protein-bound (e.g., digoxin, warfarin). Concurrent administration may produce elevated serum concentrations of both drugs.

Dosage and Administration.

Dosage. Initial dosage is usually 25 mg/day increased as tolerated to approximately 100 mg/day during the first 2 weeks. Clomipramine is usually administered in divided doses at mealtimes to reduce GI side effects. Dosage is gradually increased up to a maximum of 250 mg/day. After stabilization, the drug may be administered once per day, most commonly at bedtime to minimize daytime sedation. In children and adolescents the usual initial dosage is also 25 mg/day. The maximum daily dosage is usually 3 mg/kg or 200 mg/day, whichever is less. It is also administered in divided doses with meals. After stabilization, as with adults, the entire dose may be given at bedtime.

Administration. Clomipramine is administered orally. Owing to the long half-life of clomipramine and desmethylclomipramine, steady-state plasma levels may not be achieved until 2 to 3 weeks after a dose change. It may be appropriate therefore to wait 2 to 3 weeks between dosage adjustments.

Preparations

Clomipramine hydrochloride (*Anafranil*)
Oral capsules
25 mg, 50 mg, 75 mg

DESIPRAMINE HYDROCHLORIDE

Pharmacokinetics

Absorption. Desipramine hydrochloride is well absorbed from the GI tract with peak plasma concentrations occurring 4 to 6 hours after oral administration.

Distribution. Desipramine is distributed into breast milk.

Elimination. The elimination half-life is approximately 7 to 60 hours. Metabolism is similar to that for other TCAs.

Cautions

See Cautions under the General Statement for tricyclic antidepressants. Also notable is that Norpramin tablets contain tartrazine dye (FD & C yellow no. 5). This may cause an allergic reaction in susceptible individuals, manifested as bronchial asthma and rashes. This reaction commonly occurs in patients who are sensitive to aspirin.

Dosage and Administration

Dosage. There is a wide variation in the individual dose requirements. Dosage should be titrated to the individual's needs and tolerance. Initial dosages should be low and generally range from 25 to 75 mg/day.

Dosage is gradually increased up to a maximum of 300 mg/day in seriously ill patients. Commonly, doses of 150 to 250 mg are found to be effective. Geriatric and adolescent patients should be given lower daily dosages. Maximum antidepressant effect may require at least 3 weeks after reaching a therapeutic dose.

Administration. Desipramine hydrochloride is administered orally. Owing to its long-acting nature it may be administered in one single dose; most commonly this is given at bedtime. Patients who experience insomnia or stimulation may receive the entire daily dose in the morning.

Preparations

Desipramine hydrochloride
- Oral capsules (*Pertofrane*)
  - 25 mg, 50 mg
- Tablets (*Norpramin*)
  - 10 mg, 25 mg, 50 mg, 75 mg, 100 mg, 150 mg

DOXEPIN HYDROCHLORIDE

Pharmacokinetics

Absorption. Doxepin is well absorbed from the GI tract with peak plasma concentrations being reached within approximately 2 hours after oral administration of the drug.

Distribution. Doxepin and its active N-demethylated metabolite are distributed in breast milk.

Elimination. The plasma elimination half-life is 6 to 8 hours. The drug is metabolized via the same pathways as other TCAs. Its N-demethylated metabolite is pharmacologically active.

Cautions

See the General Statement on cautions with tricyclic antidepressants.

Dosage and Administration

Dosage. Dosage must be titrated to the individual's need and tolerance. Initial dosages should be low and generally range from 25 to 75 mg/day. Dosage is gradually adjusted upward and may range up to 300 mg/day. Children, geriatric patients, and those with an organic brain syndrome should receive lower doses. Antidepressant effects may not be seen until 3 weeks after reaching therapeutic dosages. After symptoms are controlled, the dosage should be titrated to the lowest clinically effective dose.

Administration. Doxepin hydrochloride is administered orally. Owing to its long half-life, the entire dose can be administered at one time per day. Administration at bedtime may reduce daytime sedation.

An oral concentrate is available which should be diluted in approximately 120 mL of either water, milk, or juice prior to administration. The oral concentrate is physically incompatible with many carbonated beverages. Bulk dilution and storage are not recommended.

Preparations

Doxepin hydrochloride (*Adapin, Sinequan*)
- Oral capsules
  - 10 mg, 25 mg, 50 mg, 75 mg, 100 mg, 150 mg
- Solution concentrate (*Sinequan concentrate*)
  - 10 mg/mL

IMIPRAMINE HYDROCHLORIDE, IMIPRAMINE PAMOATE

Pharmacokinetics

Absorption. The drug is completely absorbed from the GI tract with peak plasma concentrations being reached within 1 to 2 hours after oral administration and 30 minutes after IM administration.

Distribution. Imipramine and its active metabolite desipramine are distributed into breast milk.

Elimination. The plasma elimination half-life ranges from 8 to 16 hours. Imipramine is metabolized via the same pathways as other tricyclic antidepressants. Its N-monodemethylated metabolite is pharmacologically active.

Cautions

The same cautions apply to imipramine as to other TCAs. (See the General Statement on tricyclics for details.) Janimine filmtab 10- and 25-mg tablets and Tofranil-PM 100- and 125-mg tablets contain tartrazine dye (FD & C yellow no. 5). This may cause an allergic reaction in the susceptible individual. Tartrazine sensitivity is most commonly found in patients with intolerance to aspirin or asthma. Some preparations of imipramine hydrochloride contain sulfides. These may cause allergic reactions and in their most severe form anaphylaxis or severe asthmatic episodes.

Dosage and Administration

Dosage. Dosage must be titrated to the effective dose for the individual. Initial dosage usually ranges from 25 to 75 mg/day depending on the patient's general condition and severity of illness. Dosage is titrated upward to what is needed, generally not in excess of 300 mg/day. Lower doses should be used with adolescent and geriatric patients. Initial response is usually seen after 3 to 4 weeks of administration of the drug. In children under the age of 12 years dosage is usually initiated, for oral medication, at 1.5 mg/kg/day and may be increased as necessary by increments of approximately 1 mg/kg every 3 to 4 days to a maximum dosage of 5 mg/kg/day. Half this dose is usually used for the treatment of functional enuresis.

In treating children older than 6 years of age with functional enuresis, the usual initial dose of imipramine hydrochloride is 25 mg/day administered 1 hour prior to bedtime. If needed, the dose may be increased after 1 week to 50 mg per night for children younger than 12 years of age, and to 75 mg per night for children 12 years of age and older. Doses higher than 75 mg/day do not improve results. These patients are at a higher risk for side effects. For those children who tend to have their enuresis early in the night, imipramine is often administered in the late afternoon and again at bedtime.

In general, the dose of imipramine hydrochloride should not exceed 2.5 mg/kg/day in the treatment of functional enuresis. After successful treatment has been obtained, the drug should be gradually tapered and discontinued. Gradual withdrawal minimizes the likelihood of relapse. Some children who relapse may not respond to subsequent trials of imipramine.

Administration. Imipramine hydrochloride is usually administered orally; however, a parenteral form is available. Imipramine pamoate is also administered orally. Given its long half-life imipramine may be administered once a day. Usually the entire dose is given at bedtime; however, if insomnia is a problem, the entire dose may be given in the morning. In patients unwilling or unable to take imipramine orally it may be administered IM; as soon as possible, IM therapy should be switched to oral therapy.

Preparations

Imipramine hydrochloride
- Oral tablets (*Tofranil, Janimine*)
  - 10 mg, 25 mg, 50 mg

Imipramine pamoate
- Parenteral injection (*Tofranil*)
  - 12.5 mg/mL
- Oral capsules (*Tofranil-PM*)
  - 75 mg, 100 mg, 125 mg, 150 mg

MAPROTILINE HYDROCHLORIDE

Pharmacology

Maprotiline blocks the reuptake of norepinephrine at the neuronal synapse. It is also anticholinergic; however, unlike most TCAs it does not appear to influence the reuptake of serotonin. Maprotiline has a tetracyclic chemical structure; however, its clinical properties are very similar to the tricyclics.

Pharmacokinetics

Absorption. Maprotiline hydrochloride is slowly absorbed from the GI tract with peak plasma levels occurring 8 to 24 hours after a single oral dose. Steady-state plasma levels are achieved in approximately 7 days.

Distribution. Approximately 80% of maprotiline is bound to plasma proteins. Maprotiline is distributed into human breast milk.

Elimination. The plasma elimination half-life averages 51 hours with a range of 27 to 58 hours.

Metabolism. Maprotiline is metabolized in the liver to desmethylmaprotiline, a pharmacologically active compound. This is further metabolized to maprotiline-N-oxide. One-third of the ingested dose is metabolized and excreted in feces. Two-thirds is excreted in the urine as conjugated metabolites.

Uses

Maprotiline hydrochloride is used in the treatment of unipolar and bipolar major depression. It may induce manic or hypomanic episodes in patients with bipolar disorder. It appears to be as effective as the TCAs.

Cautions

Maprotiline shares the same toxicity as the TCAs (Refer to the General Statement on tricyclic antidepressants for details.) Seizures have been reported in patients taking maprotiline; many of these patients had no prior history of a seizure disorder. Maprotiline may be associated with a higher incidence of seizures than other cyclic antidepressants, but, the exact incidence remains to be determined. Seizures are more likely to occur with doses that are higher than recommended. Indeed, they usually occur in patients taking 200 mg/day or more of maprotiline, but, they have occurred in patients consuming less than that amount. To minimize the risk of seizures the lowest effective maintenance dose should be used. Likewise, other drugs known to lower seizure threshold should be avoided.

Dosage and Administration

Dosage. Dosage must be titrated to the individual's needs and tolerance. Seizure risks may be minimized by using the lowest possible dose and using a low initial dose. The initial dose is usually 25 to 75 mg/day although lower doses are used in the geriatric population. This is gradually increased, depending on tolerance, in 25-mg increments to a maximum daily dose of 100 mg/day in outpatients. In inpatients the dose may reach 225 mg/day. Many geriatric patients do well with 75 mg/day. Approximately 3 weeks are required to see the onset of antidepressant action.

Administration. Maprotiline hydrochloride is administered orally. Given its long half-life the entire dose may be administered once per day, most commonly at bedtime.

Preparations

Maprotiline hydrochloride (*Ludiomil*)
  Oral tablets
    25 mg, 50 mg, 75 mg

NORTRIPTYLINE HYDROCHLORIDE

Pharmacokinetics

Absorption. Peak plasma levels occur within 7.0 to 8.5 hours after oral administration. Optimal response to the drug usually occurs with plasma concentrations between 50 to 150 ng/mL.

Distribution. Nortriptyline is concentrated in human breast milk.

Elimination. The plasma elimination half-life ranges from 16 to 90 hours. Nortriptyline is metabolized in the same pathways as other TCAs with predominant excretion being via the kidneys.

Cautions

Nortriptyline shares the same precautions as other TCAs (See the General Statement on tricyclic antidepressants for details.) Some preparations of nortriptyline hydrochloride contain sodium bisulfite. This may produce allergic-type reactions, including anaphylaxis or life-threatening asthmatic episodes, in susceptible individuals. Such sensitivity is more common in asthmatic individuals.

Dosage and Administration

Dosage. Dosage must be titrated to an individual's need and tolerance. The usual adult dosage is 75 to 100 mg/day. Dosages greater than 100 to 150 mg are rarely necessary. When these are given, plasma concentrations should be monitored. Geriatric and adolescent patients may require lower doses than young adults.

Administration. Nortriptyline hydrochloride is administered orally. The entire dose may be given once per day, most commonly at bedtime.

Preparations

Nortriptyline hydrochloride
- Oral capsules
  - 10 mg, 25 mg (*Aventyl, Pamelor*)
  - 50 mg, 75 mg (*Pamelor*)
- Solution (*Aventyl, Pamelor*)
  - 10 mg/5 mL

PROTRIPTYLINE HYDROCHLORIDE

Pharmacokinetics

Protriptyline is completely absorbed in the GI tract with peak plasma concentrations occurring within 24 to 30 hours. Protriptyline is metabolized via the same pathways as other TCAs. Protriptyline tends to be more activating than the other TCAs.

Cautions

Protriptyline shares the same precautions as other TCAs (See the General Statement on tricyclic antidepressants for details.)

Dosage and Administration

Dosage. Dosage should be titrated to the individual's need and tolerance. Initial dosages range from 15 to 40 mg/day depending on the patient's physical status and severity of depression. Dosage should be titrated upward as needed until maximal antidepressant effect is obtained. Dosage may range up to 60 mg/day. Geriatric and adolescent patients usually will need lower doses.

Likewise, antidepressants should not be stopped abruptly but rather discontinued gradually to avoid precipitating withdrawal symptoms.

Administration. Protriptyline hydrochloride is administered orally. It may be given as a single daily dose owing to its long-acting nature.

Preparations

Protriptyline hydrochloride (*Vivactil*)
  Oral tablets
    5 mg, 10 mg

TRAZODONE HYDROCHLORIDE

Pharmacology

Complete understanding of the antidepressant action of trazodone is lacking. However, the drug is known to block reuptake of serotonin at the presynaptic neuronal membrane. This is thought to potentiate the action of serotonin at the synapse. Trazodone does not influence dopamine or norepinephrine reuptake nor does it cause release of serotonin.

With long-term administration of trazodone there is a decrease in the number of postsynaptic serotonergic and β-adrenergic receptor binding sites. This is associated with a functional increase in serotonergic activity and a reduction in the sensitivity of adenylate cyclase to stimulation by β-adrenergic agonists. This postsynaptic receptor modification may be responsible for the antidepressant effects of trazodone.

Trazodone exhibits little anticholinergic activity compared with other TCAs. Trazodone produces sedation. This varies among individuals and may represent blocking of either α-adrenergic receptors or histamine receptors. It also has an anxiolytic effect in patients who have major depression associated with anxiety.

Cardiovascular Effects. Trazodone has been associated with only minimal cardiovascular effects when compared with other TCAs. This is principally due to the absence of anticholinergic activity and catecholamine potentiating effects. Trazodone does not have substantial arrhythmogenic potential, although some arrhythmias have occurred in patients with preexisting cardiac disease.

Pharmacokinetics

Absorption. Trazodone is rapidly absorbed from the GI tract following oral administration. Increased absorption occurs with ingestion of food; however, this decreases the peak plasma concentration and lengthens the time required to reach peak plasma concentration. On an empty stomach, peak plasma concentrations are reached in approximately 1 hour, and in 2 hours after the ingestion of food. Steady state is achieved in approximately 4 days.

Distribution. Trazodone is bound approximately 95% to plasma proteins. Trazodone occurs in human breast milk in levels approximately 10% those of maternal plasma concentrations.

Uses

Major Depression. Trazodone is used in the treatment of patients with major depression with or without associated anxiety. Trazodone appears to be equally as effective an antidepressant as the TCAs. There are limited data to suggest, however, that trazodone may be more effective in treating patients with major depression and concurrent anxiety than some TCAs.

Cautions

Trazodone hydrochloride causes fewer anticholinergic side effects than those associated with the TCAs. Cardiovascular effects are also less frequent. Adverse effects appear to be dose-dependent and are more likely to occur at dosages greater than 300 mg/day. However, many patients have tolerated trazodone dosages up to 800 mg/day.

Nervous System Effects. The most frequent effects associated with trazodone therapy, occurring in 20% to 50% of all patients, are drowsiness, lightheadedness, malaise, weakness, fatigue, headache, and insomnia. Less commonly, hallucinations or delusions, disorientation, dysarthria, impaired concentration or memory, confusion, incoordination, or irritability have been reported.

Genitourinary Effects. The use of trazodone has been associated with priapism, a potential emergency. There has been permanent impairment of erectile function or impotence, or both, in some cases. Male patients should be advised that if they experience prolonged or inappropriate penile erection they should immediately discontinue the drug and consult their physician. Changes in libido, retrograde ejaculation, and impotence in men and anorgasmia in women have been associated with trazodone use.

GI Effects. The use of trazodone has been associated with nausea, vomiting, diarrhea, and flatulence.

Cardiovascular Effects. Orthostatic hypotension is the most frequent adverse cardiovascular effect, seen in 5% of patients. This is usually mild and dose-related. Trazodone may be arrhythmogenic in patients with preexisting cardiac disease.

Precautions

Because of its sedating effects trazodone may impair the ability to operate machinery or engage in activities which require mental alertness or physical coordination. Patients should be warned of this in advance, and advised that drugs such as alcohol or other CNS depressants may potentiate this effect. Likewise, patients should be advised to immediately consult a physician in the case of priapism or inappropriate or sustained erection. In overdose situations trazodone produces effects that are exaggerations of common adverse effects such as drowsiness, lethargy, nausea, vomiting, orthostatic hypotension, headache, tachycardia, and coma. Seizures and arrhythmias do not appear to be associated with trazodone overdosage. Treatment of trazodone overdosage should consist of supportive care. The stomach should be emptied by emesis or gastric lavage. The effect of activated charcoal is unknown. Hypotension should be treated appropriately, as should excessive sedation. Diuresis may help in eliminating the drug. Because of the high degree of protein binding, dialysis may not be effective in removing trazodone.

Dosage and Administration

Dosage. Dosage should be titrated to the individual's needs and tolerance. Dosage is usually begun at 100 to 150 mg/day in divided doses and increased by 50 mg every 3 to 4 days depending on the patient's need and tolerance. Outpatient dosages generally do not exceed 400 mg/day and in inpatients 600 to 800 mg/day is the usual upper limit. Full antidepressant effects may require at least 3 weeks after initiation of the drug and many patients may require longer periods. After treatment of the depressive symptoms, the lowest possible effective dose should be used.

Administration. Trazodone hydrochloride is administered orally. The drug should be administered with meals to enhance absorption. Drowsiness may be minimized by giving the larger portion of the dose at bedtime. There is some recent evidence that once-a-day dosing may be just as effective as split dosing.

Preparations

Trazodone hydrochloride
  Oral tablets
    50 mg, 100 mg (*Trialodine, Desyrel, Desyrel Dividose*)
    150 mg, 300 mg (*Desyrel Dividose*)

TRIMIPRAMINE MALEATE

Pharmacokinetics

Peak plasma concentrations of trimipramine occur approximately 2 hours after an oral dose. The plasma half-life is approximately 9 hours.

Uses

Trimipramine is used in the treatment of major depression. It appears to be equally effective as other TCAs both in treating depression and in treating enuresis.

Cautions

The same precautions observed for other TCAs should be observed for trimipramine. (See the General Statement on tricyclic antidepressants for details.)

Dosage and Administration

Dosage. Dosage should be titrated to the individual's needs and tolerance. Initial dosages usually range from 25 to 75 mg/day. Dosage is gradually titrated upward as needed and tolerated and may range up to 300 mg/day. Dosages greater than 200 mg/day are not generally recommended for outpatients. Geriatric and adolescent patients may require less than the usual adult dosage. Antidepressant effects may begin approximately 3 weeks after initiation of antidepressant treatment.

Administration. Trimipramine maleate is administered orally. When dosages do not exceed 200 mg/day, the entire daily dose can be administered once per day, most commonly at bedtime to reduce daytime sedation.

Preparations

Trimipramine maleate (*Surmontil*)
  Oral capsules
    25 mg, 50 mg, 100 mg

Monoamine Oxidase Inhibitors

GENERAL STATEMENT

In 1951 it was discovered that the new antituberculosis drug iproniazid had antidepressant properties. This led to investigations of its biochemical properties and studies of other MAOIs.

Chemistry

MAOIs are classified as either hydroxyzines or nonhydroxyzines. Hydroxyzine MAOIs include isocarboxazid and phenelzine. Nonhydroxyzine MAOIs include pargyline and tranylcypromine. More recently, MAOI's have been classified by their ability to either inhibit monoamine oxidase A or monoamine oxidase B selectively or nonselectively. The currently available MAOIs (isocarboxazid, phenelzine, and tranylcypromine) are relatively nonselective.

Pharmacology

Monoamine oxidase is an enzyme which catalyzes the oxidative deamination of epinephrine, norepinephrine, dopamine, and serotonin. The inhibition of this enzyme produces increased concentration of these amines in nerve tissue and in the liver and lungs. Tranylcypromine binds reversibly to this enzyme, whereas isocarboxazid, pargyline, and phenelzine bind irreversibly. Furthermore, there are two types of monoamine oxidase: type A, which has a preference for 5-hydroxytryptamine (5-HT) as a substrate, and type B, which has a preference for phenylthylamine. The clinical importance of these differences is not fully known. A detailed understanding of the mechanism of the antidepressant action of MAOIs is unknown. There are several working hypotheses, including an increase in free serotonin and norepinephrine within the CNS. MAOIs may produce orthostatic hypotension. This may represent a manifestation of the gradual accumulation of false neurotransmitters such as phenylethylamines in peripheral adrenergic neurons. Since these compounds are usually oxidatively deaminated in the GI tract and liver when monoamine oxidase in the GI tract and liver are inhibited, it may result in significant systemic absorption of these amines.

Octopamine may also accumulate in adrenergic neurons, as tyramine is hydroxylated to octopamine because of the inhibition of monoamine oxidase. This compound may gradually displace norepinephrine from storage granules. Stimulation of norepinephrine release may result in the release of some norepinephrine and some octopamine, the latter possibly having minimal activity at α- or β-adrenergic receptors. The gradual MAOI-induced displacement of norepinephrine from adrenergic neurons may result in a functional block of sympathetic neurotransmission. MAOIs may cause severe hypertension when foods containing large amounts of tyramine are ingested. Following absorption of tyramine there may be a rapid displacement and release of norepinephrine from adrenergic neurons resulting in severe hypertension.

The effects of MAOIs are cumulative with a period of days to months before the full onset of antidepressant activity become manifest. There is some evidence that the antidepressant effect manifests when platelet monoamine oxidase is inhibited by at least 85%. Measuring these levels of inhibition is not yet clinically done.

Uses

MAOIs are used for the symptomatic management of patients with depression. In particular, individuals with so-called atypical depression may preferentially respond to MAOIs. These individuals exhibit reactivity of mood, weight gain, hypersomnia, hypersensitivity to rejection, and carbohydrate craving. MAOIs are helpful with agoraphobia. Many reserve the use of MAOIs for patients who have responded poorly to heterocyclic antidepressants. Some patients preferentially respond to one MAOI and not to others.

Cautions

Hypertensive Crisis. Hypertensive crisis is the most serious adverse reaction associated with MAOI therapy and may be fatal.

It is characterized by severe headache, nausea or vomiting, sweating, neck stiffness or soreness, and mydriasis with or without visual disturbances. Intracranial hemorrhage, which may be fatal, has been reported to occur in some patients during hypertensive crisis.

MAOIs should be immediately discontinued if a hypertensive crisis occurs, and the individual treated with an α-adrenergic blocking agent such as phentolamine. This should be administered via intravenous (IV) injection. The usual adult dose is 2 to 5 mg. This will lower blood pressure and subsequently result in resolution of the headache. Fever may be managed by external cooling, if necessary.

Other Adverse Effects. Most other effects are dose related and resolve or diminish with reduction in dosage. Frequently associated side effects include restlessness, insomnia, anorexia, constipation, nausea and vomiting, dry mouth, blurred vision, urinary retention, impotence, drowsiness, orthostatic hypotension, headache, rash, dizziness, and weakness. Orthostatic hypotension is a common dose-related adverse effect of MAOIs. Drug increases should be more gradual in those patients who show orthostatic hypotension during initiation of drug treatment. If orthostatic hypotension persists, or is severe, possible responses include dose reduction, discontinuation of therapy, the use of support stockings, additional salt in the diet, or the use of the mineral corticoid fludrocortisone (Florinef).

Other side effects include increased perspiration, urinary frequency, flushing, weight gain associated with an increase in appetite, numbness, paresthesias, tremor and myoclonic jerks, hyperreflexia, and muscle spasms. Hypomania and mania have occurred in some patients. There have been reports of dependence of tranylcypromine developing in individuals treated with therapeutic dosages substantially larger than the usual. Many of these patients had a prior history of substance abuse.

Precautions and Contraindications. Blood pressure should be carefully monitored during initiation of therapy to evaluate orthostatic hypotension or a pressor response. Clinical signs also helpful for the determination of hypertension would include headache or palpitations. Patients receiving MAOIs should be warned against eating foods high in tyramine; certain alcoholic beverages are also rich in tyramine. Likewise, patients should be cautioned not to use any over-the-counter cough, cold, or weight-reducing preparation unless under the supervision of a physician; many of these preparations contain pressor agents. Tables 2–2 and 2–3 list the restricted foods and medications for patients taking MAOIs. The patient should be advised to contact his or her physician and, if need be, proceed to an emergency room if signs of hypertension develop.

Depressed patients are at an increased risk for suicide. Appropriate precautions, including hospitalization, if necessary, should be maintained during the period of time at risk for suicide. In particular, during the period of initiation of drug treatment individuals may be at risk for suicide. Reliance on drug therapy alone to prevent suicide is often hazardous. MAOIs may suppress internal pain in patients with myocardial ischemia, and therefore patients with angina or coronary artery disease should be warned about overexertion. Caution should be used in patients with impaired renal function to avoid accumulation of MAOI in the plasma of these patients. Liver function (bilirubin, serum alkaline phosphatase, serum aminotransferases) should be monitored periodically to detect possible hepatic damage from MAOIs.

Pregnancy, Fertility, and Lactation. The safety of MAOIs during pregnancy has not been established. The drugs should be used during pregnancy only when the potential benefits justify the potential risks.

Tranylcypromine has been shown to cross the placenta in animals. In addition, tranylcypromine is distributed into the milk of lactating animals. It is, however, unknown if MAOIs are distributed into human milk. MAOIs should be used with caution in nursing women.

Toxicity

Manifestations. Signs of overdose are extensions of common adverse reactions. In mild overdose situations drowsiness, dizziness, ataxia, headache, insomnia, restlessness, anxiety, and irritability are common. Severe overdosage may include mental confusion, incoherence, tachycardia, rapid and irregular pulse, hyper- or hypotension, coma, seizures, respiratory depression, hyper- or hyporeflexia, fever, diaphoresis, precordial pain, and shock. Some patients may develop twitching, myoclonic fibrillation of skeletal muscles, hyperpyrexia, trismus, or opisthotonos.

Table 2–2.
Dietary Precautions for Patients Taking Monoamine Oxidase Inhibitor (MAOI) Antidepressants*

Foods That Must Be Avoided	Foods That May Be Consumed With Caution†
Cheese	Avocado
Smoked or pickled meats, fish, or poultry; caviar; game	Cottage cheese, cream cheese
Nonfresh meat, nonfresh livers	Raspberries
Chianti and vermouth wines	Fresh-frozen meat, liver, poultry, fish
Distilled spirits to which red wine has been added	Distilled spirits
Broad bean pods (fava or Italian broad beans; Chinese pea pods)	Soy sauce
Banana peel	String beans, lima beans, dry beans
Meat extracts used as a base for soup, gravy, and sauces (bouillon, consommé, Bovril, marmite)	Red and white wines (except Chianti and vermouth)
Brewer's yeast and yeast extracts	Port, sherry
Sausage, corned beef	Baker's yeast
sauerkraut	Bacon
Beer, ale, with or without alcohol	Yogurt from unpasteurized milk
	Cream from unpasturized milk
	Miso soup or soup stock

*These food precautions should be followed for 2 weeks after stopping the MAOI.

†"Consumed with caution" means small servings (1/2 cup, 4 oz, 120 mL, or less). Any food, especially a high-protein food, should not be consumed unless freshly prepared after brief shelf storage. Any food that previously caused illness or unpleasant symptoms should be avoided.

Table 2–3.
Medication Precautions for Patients Taking Monoamine Oxidase Inhibitor (MAOI) Antidepressants*

Over-the-counter preparations	For colds, nasal, sinus, or throat congestion; coughs; hay fever; nasal or sinus allergy; or asthma (tablets, capsules, drops, sprays, and inhalant)
Meperidine (Demerol)	For weight reduction or appetite control or suppression
Dextromethorphan	Often used as a cough suppressant
Cocaine, amphetamines	"Uppers" or "pep pills"
Epinephrine	Often added to local anesthetics, as in dental procedures
Other antidepressants	Unless approved by a physician

*Medications, drugs and proprietary preparations of any kind should only be taken after first consulting a physician. These medication precautions should be followed for 2 weeks after stopping the MAOI.

Agitation or hyperactivity may occur. Signs and symptoms of acute overdose usually resolve within 3 to 4 days but may persist for up to 2 weeks in some patients. Careful observation of patients for at least 1 week after overdose is generally recommended.

Treatment. Treatment of an MAOI overdose involves symptomatic supportive care. During the immediate postingestion period the stomach should be emptied by gastric lavage. During the acute overdose period it is important to remember that many drugs interact with MAOIs. Therefore, conservative measures are usually used to treat clinical problems. For example, hyperthermia is treated with external cooling; hypotension is usually treated by volume expansion. Pressor amines such as norepinephrine may be of limited value and may result in hypertension when used with MAOIs because of potentiation by MAOIs. In general, the direct-acting amines (epinephrine and norepinephrine) are less dangerous than the indirect amines (e.g., amphetamine, ephedrine, and tyramine).

Liver function should be evaluated at the time of overdose and for 4 to 6 weeks following recovery. During the overdose period, if hyperactivity or agitation occur, administration of a phenothiazine may be necessary.

Drug Interactions

Food. Hypertensive crises have occurred following ingestion of foods containing large amounts of either tryptophan or tyramine in patients receiving MAOIs. In general, patients should be instructed to avoid foods in which there is aging or breakdown of protein. In addition, excessive amounts of caffeine may precipitate a hypertensive crisis. (See Table 2–2 for a detailed listing of foods to be avoided.)

Antidepressants Agents. Concomitant administration of TCAs and MAOIs has been reported to produce hyperpyretic states, seizures, and death. However, this usually occurs following overdosage or parenteral administration of one or both of these drugs. Following oral administration of both drugs in therapeutic ranges, hyperpyrexia, hypertension, tachycardia, confusion, and seizures have been reported. This reaction is distinct from the hypertensive crises that may occur with other MAOI interactions (Table 2–4). Some manufacturers have recommended that at least 1 to 2 weeks elapse before switching from a TCA to an MAOI or from one MAOI to another. Further, they recommend that the MAOI be initiated at one-half the usual dosage and maintained at that dosage for at least 1 week.

Similarly, many recommend allowing 1 week to elapse after discontinuation of an MAOI and the administration of a TCA. The two classes of drugs should only be used together when the potential benefits clearly exceed the potential risks to the patient. If the two classes of drugs are used together, large doses should be avoided if possible. It is also preferable to either start the drugs together or start the TCA first: avoid adding TCAs to a patient already started on MAOIs. In addition, for those patients with suicidal ideation, the clinician should consider the potential lethality of the two drugs when used in combination.

Sympathomimetic and Catecholamine-Releasing Agents. Some patients may be at greater risk for an exaggerated response to the effects of sympathomimetic agents during MAOI therapy. Those compounds which include amphetamines and peripherally acting agents such as over-the-counter cold, hay fever, and weight-reducing preparations (e.g., ephedrine, phenylpropanolamine) should not be administered concurrently with an MAOI.

CNS Depressants and Opiates. MAOI's may potentiate or be additive with the effect of alcohol, opiates, other analgesics, and barbiturates. These compounds should be administered with caution to avoid sedation or hypotension; a reduction in dosage may be necessary. Meperidine should not be used in patients receiving MAOIs since there have been reports of excitation, sweating, hyperpyrexia, hypertension, rigidity, and death.

Buspirone. Because of reports of elevations in blood pressure in patients receiving MAOIs and busiprone concomitantly, it is recommended that MAOIs not be used with buspirone. It is suggested to wait 10 days following discontinuation of an MAOI inhibitor before the administration of busiprone.

ISOCARBOXAZID

Uses

Isocarboxazid is commonly used in patients who have failed to respond to other antidepressant therapy, especially heterocyclics or ECT. It is used for the symptomatic treatment of depression in such patients. Because the response to MAOIs is highly variable, individuals who do not respond to one particular preparation may respond to other drugs in this class.

It is difficult to establish a cause-effect relationship for interactions between MAOIs and other substances. Firstly, MAOIs act by forming an irreversible combination with the enzyme monoamine oxidase, which is continuously being synthesized in the body. Depending on the different dose and duration of treatment, the level of monoamine oxidase inhibition may persist to some degree for up to 2 weeks after treatment ceases. Secondly, the amine composition of foodstuffs is also variable and unpredictable. For example, cheeses with an identical appearance may vary 100-fold in tyramine content, and the unpredictability in the occurrence of adverse effects, has contributed to the unpopularity of the MAOIs as therapeutic agents. The interactions with MAOIs fall into two categories: an exacerbation or prolongation of the normally occurring effects of the drug (sedation or coma caused by alcohol, anes-

Table 2–4.
Drug Interactions With Monoamine Oxidase Inhibitors (MAOIs)

Combination	Interaction Effects	Mechanism/ Comments	Clinical Significance
Antibiotics (phenelzine + sulfonamides)	↑ Both drugs' plasma (levels and side effects (ataxia, vertigo, tinnitus, muscle pain, parethesias)	? Additional acetylation of both drugs	?
Anesthetics	Anesthesia may be potentiated Hypertensive crisis (in epinephrine, norepinephrine preperations)	Potentiate action at central receptor site	Yes
Anticholinergics, antiparkinsonian drugs	MAOI potentiates the action of coadministered agents	? Mechanism Discontinue MAOI prior to elective surgery ↓ Dosages of anticholinergic agents	
Anticoagulants (coumarin)	Potentiate anticoagulant action	Inhibition of metabolism	Yes
Antihypertensive drugs	Antagonize hypotensive effect	May inhibit amine uptake	Yes
Guanethidine, methyldopa	Signs of central stimulation (with methyldopa)	Avoid such combinations Phentolamine (Regitine) should be used in such cases	
β-Adrenergic blockers (e.g., propranolol)	Severe hypertensive crisis	Contraindication in combination; otherwise, with very low dose of propranolol β-Receptor blockade caused by unopposed α-adrenergic activity Bradycardia: 2 elderly cases reported	Yes

Reserpine and rauwolfia alkaloids	↑ Hypertension and central excitation (theoretically)	Reserpine depletes intracellular catecholamines Case report only Do not give reserpine to patients stabilized on MAOIs (i.e., use reserpine prior to MAOI)	?
Appetite suppressants, amphetamines, other sympathomimetics (e.g, bronchodilators, nasal decongestants, hypertensive agents)	Hypertensive episodes, cardiac arrhythmias, hyperpyrexia, agitation, hyperkinesis, headache, opisthotonos, convulsions	↓ Metabolism of sympathomimetic amines	Yes
Indirect-acting sympathomimetics (more dangerous): amphetamine (methamphetamine), cyclopentamine, ephedrine, pseudoephedrine, levodopa, dopamine, mephentermine, phentermine, metaraminol, methylphenidate, Phenylpropanolamine, Tyramine		Conflicting results: some combination reports without problems Phenelzine, tranylcypromine, and furazolidone (furoxone) are more dangerous? (amphetamine-like or sensitive MAOI) Should avoid combination or let 2-wk elapse after stopping MAOI	
Direct-acting sympathomimetics (less dangerous): norepinephrine, epinephrine, phenylephrine, isoproterenol, methoxamine		Treatment: α-Blocker: phentolamine for hypertension β-blocker: for tachycardia and arrhythmia Chlorpromazine for CNS effects	

(Continued.)

Table 2–4 (cont.).

Combination	Interaction Effects	Mechanism/ Comments	Clinical Significance
Aspartame and carbohydrate load	Headache, ↑ blood pressure (?) flushing, sweating	CNS tyrosine level One case report	?
Barbiturates, sedative-hypnotics	↑ Barbiturate and sedative-hypnotic effects	? Inhibition of metabolism Case reports	Yes
Carbamazepine (Tegretol)	Possible effects as TCA + MAOI	No clinical report Manufacturer lists under contraindications	?
Caffeine or other xanthine	Hyperexcitability reactions	Mechanism? Stopping or reducing caffeine intake; no specific treatment required	?
CNS depressants	↑ CNS sedation	Potentiation at receptor site	Yes
Dextromethorphan	Nausea, coma, hypotension, hyperpyrexia, death	Mechanism? Case report suspected evidence of interaction	?
Doxapram (Dopram)	Hypertension, arrhythmias	Caution with concomitant use	?
Ethanol	↑ Sedation		
	↑ Alcohol intoxication Hypertensive crisis	MAOIs alcohol metabolism Some alcoholic beverages, (Chianti, other red wines, imported beer) may contain large amounts of tyramine Alcohol ↑ central catecholamine synthesis and release	Yes

		No tyramine-containing acoholic beverages (gin, vodka, whiskey, white wines, etc.)	
Food with high tyramine content (e.g, broad beans, red wines (chianti), yeast extract, some imported beers, chicken or beef liver, caviar, pickled herring, fermented sausage [e.g., bologna, pepperoni, salami, summer sausage], overripe avocados and various cheeses [e.g., Brie, camembert, Cheddar, Emmentaler, Gruyère, Mozzarella, Parmesan, Romano, Roquefort, Stilton]	Hypertensive crisis (cheese reaction): pounding headache, flushing, photophobia, dilated pupils, choking sensation, nausea, vomiting hypertension, diaphoresis, chest pain, tachycardia or bradycardia, palpitation	MAOIs inhibit metabolism of tyramine and other pressor amines Food with high tyramine content must be avoided Symptoms onset: usually about 2 hr after ingestion of food high in tyramine MAOI effects may linger for 2–4 wk after the drug is discontinued *Management:* antihistamine (diphenhydramine 25 mg) for headache *Mild cases:* Oral (sublingual) mifedipine 10–20 mg *Severe cases:* phentolamine 2–5 slow IV; Diazoxide 50–100 mg rapid IV; sodium nitroprusside 50–100 mg in IV glucose External cooling	Yes
Hypoglycemic drugs (insulin, sulfonylureas)	MAOIs enhance or prolong hypoglycemic responses to both insulin and sulfonylureas	Stimulation of endogenous insulin secretion and inhibition of gluconeogenesis (compensatory adrenergic response)	Yes

(Continued.)

Table 2–4 (cont.).

Combination	Interaction Effects	Mechanism/ Comments	Clinical Significance
		Delayed onset of interaction (several weeks) for insulin but rapid onset for sulfonylureas	
Levodopa	See Sympathomimetics	Use of decraboxylase inhibitor (e.g., carbidopa) with levodopa apparently prevents hypertensive reactions MAO type B inhibitor selegiline (Eldepryl) + levodopa + carbidopa → no hypertensive reactions	Yes
Lithium	↑ MAOI antidepressive effect Chronic coadministration → tardive dyskinesia (?)	Mechanism ? Helpful for treatment of refractory depression	Yes
Local anesthetics with vasoconstrictors (dental) (see Sympathomimetics)	Hypertension	Postsynaptic denervation hypersensitivity Controversial results Suitable alternatives: levonordefrin, lidocaine, mepivacaine	Yes

MAOIs (switching from other MAOIs to tranylcypromine	Hypertensive reaction	? Amphetamine-MAOI interaction At least 1–2 wks should elapse between 2 different MAOIs, espcially when the second drug is tranylcypromine	Yes
Mazindol (Teronac) (anti-obesity agent) (see also Sympathomimetics)	↑ Pressor action of catecholamines	Potentiates intrinsic sympathetic activity Avoid combination At least 1 mo should elaspe between between stopping 1 agent and starting the other	Yes
Methotrimeprazine (levoprome)	Fatal reaction Case reports	Mechanism ?	?
Narcotic analgesics (e.g., Meperidine [Demerol], Morphine)	Excitation, rigidity, coma, hypo- or hypertension, hyperpyrexia Prolongation of narcotic effects may be fatal	Probably serotonin-mediated Rapid onset (about 1–2 min) of effects Avoid MAOI + meperidine Other narcotics (e.g., morphine) may be given cautiously, and in reduced dose Management: chlorpromazine, nalorphine, prednisolone are of value	Yes
Neuroleptics (esp. phenothiazine)	Potentiate hypotensive and extrapyramidal reactions	Mechanism ? MAOI may inhibit metabolism of phenothiazine	?

(Continued.)

Table 2–4 (cont.).

Combination	Interaction Effects	Mechanism/ Comments	Clinical Significance
	Prolong and enhance anticholinergic reactions	Controversial report, some combination reports—decreased side effects of both drugs and protection against tyramine-induced hypertensive crises	
Steroids	Counteract orthostatic hypotension induced by MAOI	Mechanism ? Fludrocortisone: 0.3–0.6 mg/day may allow MAOI treatment to continue	?
Succinycholine (Annectine, Quelicin)	Prolonged apnea	↓ Plasma pseudocholinesterase Case reports: phenelzine (Nardil) only	Yes
Theophyline (oxtriphyline) and xanthine bronchodilator	Anxiety, palpitations, tachycardia	Mechanism ?	?
Thiazide diuretics	Enhanced hypotensive effects	Mechanism ?	Yes
TCAs (See Table 1–1)			
Tryptophan	Acute behaviorial and neurologic toxicity, e.g., myoclonus, hypomanic episode, agitation, delirium Useful for treatment of refractory depresssion	Mechanisms ? May be due to stimulation of serotonergic system Start tryptophan from a lower dose such as 0.25 or 0.5 g and gradually titrate upward	?

thetics, or opiate analgesics; central anticholinergic toxicity due to TCAs), or a hypertensive crisis attributable to the release and potentiation of catecholamines. The consequences of the hypertensive reaction are also variable.

Food. Hypertensive crises have occurred following ingestion of foods containing large amounts of either tryptophan or tyramine in patients receiving MAOIs. In general, patients should be instructed to avoid foods in which there is aging or breakdown of protein. In addition, excessive amounts of caffeine may precipitate a hypertensive crisis. (See Table 1–2 for a detailed listing of foods to be avoided.)

Antidepressants Agents. The most commonly encountered adverse effect of MAOIs is the production of postural hypotension, which may in fact, be potentiated in some patients receiving TCAs in combination with MAOIs. It is theoretically possible that combined tricyclic-MAOI therapy could provoke a higher incidence of hypertensive reactions. Clinically, the combination has been reported to produce hyperpyretic states, seizures, and death. However, this usually occurs following overdosage or parenteral administration of one or both of these drugs. Following oral administration of both drugs in therapeutic ranges, hyperpyrexia, hypertension, tachycardia, confusion, and seizures have been reported. Based on controlled studies and clinical observation, this combined TCA-MAOI therapy does not appear to be associated with a high risk of hypertensive or hyperpyretic crises.

Some manufacturers have recommended that at least 1 to 2 weeks elapse before switching from a TCA to an MAOI or from one MAOI to another, especially when the second drug is tranylcypromine. Abruptly changing treatment from another MAOI to tranylcypromine has been reported to produce a potentially fatal hypertensive reaction. There is substantial case report evidence for hazards in adding a TCA to an established course of MAOI. It still seems best to begin combined MAOI-TCA treatment by starting the two drugs at the same time, the combination commonly recommended in the clinical literature, allowing first a week off either type of drug, then starting both together within the same 24-hour period at low dosage, and gradually increasing the dosages of both together to a maximum of half that used with single-drug treatment. The two classes of drugs should only be used together when the potential benefits clearly exceed the potential risks to the patient and, for those patients with suicidal ideation, the clinician should consider the potential lethality of the two drugs when used in combination. Since as serious and even fatal outcomes have been reported when MAOIs have been combined with either clomipramine or fluoxetine, it is essential to avoid the combinations of MAOIs with any of the serotonin reuptake-inhibiting drugs. Otherwise, sufficient time must elapse between administering these two classes of drugs.

Sympathomimetic and Catecholamine-Releasing Agents. Some patients may be at greater risk for unexaggerated response to the effects of sympathomimetic agents during MAOI therapy. These compounds, which include amphetamines and tyramine and peripherally acting agents such as over-the-counter nose drops, cold remedies, nasal decongestants, cough syrups, bronchodilators, diet pills, and hay fever preparations (e.g., ephedrine, phenylpropanolamine), should not be administered concurrently with an MAOI. The current epidemic of cocaine abuse indicates the necessity to specifically warn the patient against the use of cocaine while taking an MAOI. With the combined therapy, hypertensive reaction and acute transient psychosis have been reported.

CNS Depressants. MAOIs may potentiate or be additive with the effect of alcohol, barbiturates, benzodiazepines, chloral hydrate, opiates, and other analgesics. These compounds should be administered with caution to avoid sedation or hypotension; a reduction in dosage may be necessary. Meperidine should not be used in patients receiving MAOIs since there have been reports of excitation, sweating, hyperpyrexia, profound hypotension or dramatic hypertension, rigidity, and death.

Cardiac and Antihypertensive Drugs. There are a number of potential interactions between MAOIs and antihypertensive agents. An MAOI-treated patient who is started on guanethidine or clonidine may experience a hypertensive reaction followed by severe hypotension. Methyldopa can also provoke a hypertensive reaction in a patient receiving an MAOI. Hydralazine is likely to produce pronounced tachycardia and possibly elevated blood pressure in a patient receiving MAOI antidepressants. Any vasodilator may tend to enhance the hypotensive reaction—the most common unwanted effect of MAOI antidepressants. If a neuroleptic is necessary in conjunction with therapy with MAOI antidepressants, piperazine phenothiazines such as trifluoperazine or the butyrophenone haloperidol are clearly the safest drugs with the least likelihood of producing a hypotensive reaction.

Busiprone. Because of reports of elevations in blood pressure in patients receiving MAOIs and busiprone concomitantly, it is recommended currently that MAOIs not be used with buspirone. A 10-day wait is suggested following discontinuation of an MAOI and the administration of busiprone.

Miscellaneous. Concurrent administration of levodopa and an MAOI may produce pronounced CNS stimulation and hypertension. A similar reaction may occur with the respiratory center stimulant doxapram. It is generally preferable to delay elective surgery for 1 to 2 weeks after discontinuing an MAOI. Several drug interactions between MAOIs and anesthetics have been reported. Halothane and enflurance have both been reported to produce muscle stiffness and hyperpyrexia in MAOI-treated patients. Succinylcholine and related muscle relaxants may have their paralytic effect potentiated and prolonged as the result of MAOI treatment.

Adequate patient education is essential to the safer use of these drugs. The patient must be aware of the name and the nature of the drug he or she is taking and its potential to interact with foods and medications. Additionally, the patient should understand what symptoms may indicate an interaction, such as unexpected drowsiness or sudden severe throbbing headache, etc.

Cautions

Isocarboxazid is as toxic as other MAOIs. Because of this patients should be informed of the potential adverse risks, in particular hypertensive crisis. The same precautions and contraindications hold true for isocarboxazid as for all MAOIs.

Dosage and Administration

Dosage. Dosage must be titrated to the individual's requirements and tolerance. The goal is to use the lowest possible clinically effective dosage. Side effects are dose-dependent. The clinical response to the antidepressant effect is gradual and usually occurs over a period of approximately 3 to 4 weeks, although in some patients some relief may be seen in the first week of therapy. If no signs of a beneficial response are seen after 4 weeks, further improvement in depressive symptomatology with continued drug use is unlikely.

The usual initiating dose for treatment of depression is 30 mg/day given in divided doses or as a single dose.

Administration. Isocarboxazid is administered orally.

Preparations

Isocarboxazid (*Marplan*)
Oral tablets
10 mg

PHENELZINE SULFATE

Pharmacology

The principle pharmacologic effects of phenelzine are similar to those of other hydrazine-derived MAOIs. Phenelzine is used for the treatment of depression. The drug is generally reserved for those who have been refractory to either ECT or heterocyclic antidepressants, or for patients with atypical depressions. This drug has been used in combination with TCAs for the management of patients who have been refractory when treated with other antidepressant agents (See the General Statement regarding MAOIs.)

The patient response to antidepressants is individual; patients may respond preferentially to one antidepressant in this class as opposed to another.

Cautions

Phenelzine shares the risks of other drugs in this class. Signs of toxicity (including those associated with overdose) and drug interactions (including those with certain foods) are the same as for other drugs in this category.

Dosage and Administration

Dosage. Dosage should be titrated to the lowest effective dose for the individual. The antidepressant response is gradual and may require 3 to 4 weeks for therapeutic effect. The usual initial adult dosage is 15 mg given one to two times a day. Dosage should be increased to at least 60 mg/day as rapidly as tolerated. Dosages up to, or in excess of, 90 mg/day may be required in some patients.

Administration. Phenelzine sulfate is administered orally.

Preparations

Phenelzine sulphate (*Nardil*)
Oral tablets
15 mg

TRANYLCYPROMINE SULFATE

Pharmacology

The principle pharmacologic effects of tranylcypromine are the same as for the other nonhydrazine MAOIs. Many believe that tranylcypromine may produce greater CNS stimulation than other MAOIs. This may be related to the close structural similarity between tranylcypromine and amphetamine.

Pharmacokinetics

The onset of action of tranylcypromine may be more rapid than that of hydrazine-type MAOIs. In addition, tranylcypromine does not produce as prolonged an inhibition of the enzyme following drug discontinuation. The drug is excreted within approximately 24 hours.

Uses

Tranylcypromine is used to treat severe depression. The patient response is variable. Some individuals who do not respond to one drug in this class may respond to another.

Cautions

Tranylcypromine is similar to other MAOIs in terms of toxicity, drug interactions, and interactions with foods rich in tryptophan or tyramine. Patients should be cautioned of the need for dietary restrictions and discretion in the use of over-the-counter cough and cold preparations (see Table 2–3).

Dosage and Administration

Dosage. The dosage of tranylcypromine must be titrated to the individual's needs using the lowest clinically effective dosage. Therapeutic onset is gradual and occurs over approximately 3 to 4 weeks. The usual dosage is 30 mg/day, usually given in two divided doses. If no therapeutic response occurs after the first 2 to 3 weeks, the dosage may be increased by 10 mg/day at 1- to 3-

week intervals, up to 60 mg/day. Side effects are dose related and are more likely to occur in dosages in excess of 30 mg/day. Once an adequate response has been achieved, the dosage should be lowered to the lowest clinically effective dose.

Administration. Tranylcypromine sulfate is administered orally.

Preparations

Tranylcypromine sulfate (*Parnate*)
Oral tablets
10 mg

Serotonin Reuptake Inhibitors

GENERAL STATEMENT

Pharmacology/Mechanism of Action

Serotonin reuptake inhibitors (SRIs), also called selective serotonin reuptake inhibitors (SSRIs), are oral antidepressant agents that are chemically unrelated to tricyclic, heterocyclic, or other antidepressants. Their mechanism of action is presumed to be related to their potent and selective inhibition of neuronal uptake of serotonin in the brain. These agents have weak effects on norepinephrine and dopamine uptake. Because of their limited affinity for α_1-, α_2-, β-adrenergic, benzodiazepine, dopamine-2, GABA, histamine, and muscarinic receptors, these agents also are free of many of the side effects that have been associated with other psychotropic medications, such as anticholinergic, sedative, and cardiovascular effects.

Pharmacokinetics

Fluoxetine has a half-life for the parent drug, and its active metabolite (norfluoxetine) ranges from 48 to 216 hours. The steady state of fluoxetine is reached within 28 to 35 days and the primary route of elimination is via the liver. Fluvoxamine has a half-life that ranges from 13.6 to 15.6 hours and reaches its steady state in about 7 days. The primary route of elimination is via the kidneys. Paroxetine has a half-life of 21 hours and achieves its steady state in approximately 10 hours. The primary routes of elimination are via the kidneys and the liver. Sertraline has a half-life that ranges from 26 to 65 hours and reaches its steady state in 7 days. The primary routes of elimination are equally divided between the kidneys and the liver.

Uses

Fluoxetine is indicated for the treatment of depression and obsessive-compulsive disorder. Non-U.S. Food and Drug Administration (FDA) approved uses include the treatment of bulimia nervosa (at dosages of 60 to 80 mg/day) and obesity (at dosages of 20 to 60 mg/day).

Fluvoxamine is indicated in the treatment of obsessive-compulsive disorder and is being studied in the treatment of depression.

Paroxetine is indicated in the treatment of depression.

Sertraline is indicated in the treatment of depression and under investigation in the treatment of obsessive-compulsive disorder.

Cautions

Contraindications. SRIs are contraindicated in patients with a known sensitivity to these agents. They are also contraindicated in patients taking a MAOI or within 14 days of discontinuing an MAOI. Fluvoxamine is contraindicated in patients taking terfenadine or astemizole.

Renal Impairment. In patients with impaired renal function, increased concentrations of paroxetine occur. In patients with a Ccr <30 ml/min, levels are four times those of normal subjects. When Ccr is 30 to 60 ml/min, there is a twofold increase in paroxetine plasma levels. With chronic use of fluoxetine in patients with severely impared renal function, accumulation of fluoxetine or its metabolites may occur. While renal excretion of sertraline is a minor route of elimination, caution should be used in patients with severe renal impairment.

Hepatic Impairment. In patients with impaired hepatic function, the elimination half-life of SRIs may be prolonged. The initial dosages should be lower and upward titration slower. Dosing may be less frequent.

Activation of Mania/Hypomania. Activation of mania/hypomania may occur. During premarketing testing, hypomania or mania occurred in approximately 0.4% of sertraline-treated patients. Hypomania occurred in approximately in 1.0% of paroxetine–treated unipolar patients compared with 1.1% of active-control and 0.3% of placebo-treated unipolar patients. In a subset of patients classified as bipolar, the rate of manic episodes was 2.2% for paroxetine and 11.6% for the combined active-control groups. Activation of mania/hypomania has also been reported in a small proportion of patients with affective disorders that were treated with other marketed antidepressants. As with all antidepressants, SRIs should be used cautiously in patients with a history of mania.

Suicide. The possibility of a suicide attempt is inherent in depression and may persist until significant remission occurs. Close supervision of high-risk patients should accompany initial drug therapy. Prescriptions for SRIs should be written for the smallest quantity of tablets consistent with good patient management to reduce the risk of overdose.

Concomitant Illness. Clinical experience with SRIs in patients with certain concomitant systemic illness is limited. Caution is advisable in using SRIs in patients with diseases or conditions that could affect metabolism or hemodynamic responses.

Increased plasma concentrations of some SRIs may occur in patients with severe renal impairment (creatinine clearance <30 ml/min.) or severe hepatic impairment. A lower starting dosage should be used in such patients (see *Dosage and Administration*). Sertraline is extensively metabolized by the liver. In subjects with mild, stable cirrhosis of the liver, the clearance of sertraline was decreased, thus increasing the elimination half-life. A lower or less frequent dose should be used in patients with cirrhosis. Since sertraline is extensively metabolized, excretion of unchanged drug in urine is a minor route of elimination. However, until the pharmacokinetics of sertraline have been studied in patients with renal impairment and until adequate numbers of patients with severe renal impairment have been evaluated during chronic treatment with sertraline, this drug should be used with caution in such patients.

Interference with Cognitive and Motor Performance. Any psychoactive drug may impair judgement, thinking, or motor skills. Although SRIs have not been shown to impair psychomotor performance, patients should be cautioned about operating hazardous machinery, including automobiles, until they are reasonably certain that the medication does not affect their ability to engage in such activities.

Concomitant Medication. Patients should be advised to inform their physician if they are taking, or plan to take, any prescription or over-the-counter drugs, since there is a potential for interactions.

Long-Term Use. Long-term efficacy of SRIs has not been fully established. Studies suggest paroxetine is effective for up to one year. Studies also support the efficacy of sertraline for up to 16 weeks in depression and 13 weeks in obsessive–compulsive disorder. If SRIs are utilized for prolonged periods, continued efficacy and indication should be assessed in the individual patient.

Drug Interactions

Drugs Highly Bound to Plasma Protein. Sertraline and paroxetine are highly protein bound. If administered with other medications that are also highly protein bound, the free concentration of either drug may increase and result in adverse effects to the patient. Because paroxetine is highly bound to plasma protein, administration of paroxetine to a patient taking another drug that is highly protein bound may cause increased free concentrations of the other drug, potentially resulting in adverse events. Conversely, adverse effects could result from displacement of paroxetine by other highly bound drugs. Because sertraline is tightly bound to plasma protein, the administration of sertraline (sertraline hydrochloride) to a patient taking another drug that is tightly bound to protein (e.g., warfarin, digitoxin) may cause a shift in plasma concentrations, potentially resulting in an adverse effect. Conversely, adverse effects may result from displacement of protein-bound sertraline by other tightly bound drugs.

Microsomal Enzymes. Sertraline has the ability to induce hepatic micosomal enzyme; however, the clinical effect may be minimal.

Coadministration of paroxetine with drugs that are metabolized by the cytochrome P450IID6 isoenzyme, such as phenothiazines, some antidepressants, Type IC antiarrhythmics, or drugs that inhibit this enzyme, such as quinidine, should be done with caution to avoid toxicity. Fluvoxamine is a weak inhibitor of this isoenzyme.

Concomitant use of SRIs with drugs metabolized by cytochrome P450IID6 has not been formally studied but may require lower doses than usually prescribed for either SRI or the other drug. Many drugs, including most antidepressants (SRIs and many tricyclics), are metabolized by the cytochrome P450 isozyme P450IID6. In most patients (>90%), this P450IID6 isozyme is saturated early during paroxetine dosing. Like other agents that are metabolized by P450IID6, paroxetine may significantly inhibit the activity of this isozyme. Therefore, coadministration of SRIs with other drugs that are metabolized by this isozyme, including certain antidepressants (e.g., nortriptyline, amitriptyline, imipramine, desipramine, and fluoxetine), phenothiazines (e.g., thioridazine), and type 1C antiarrhythmics (e.g., propafenone, flecainide, and encainide), or that inhibit this enzyme (e.g., quinidine) should be approached with caution. At steady state, when the P450IID6 pathway is essentially saturated, paroxetine clearance is governed by alternative P450 isozymes, which unlike P450IID6, show no evidence of saturation.

Tryptophan

An interaction between SRIs and tryptophan may occur when they are coadministered. Adverse experiences, consisting primarily of headache, nausea, sweating, and dizziness, have been reported when tryptophan was administered to such patients. Consequently, concomitant use of SRIs with tryptophan is not recommended.

MAOIs

Cases of serious reactions have been reported in patients receiving SRIs in combination with a monoamine oxidase inhibitor (MAOI). The symptoms have included mental status changes, such as memory changes, confusion, and irritability, chills, pyrexia, and muscle rigidity. In patients receiving SRIs in combination with a monoamine oxidase inhibitor (MAOI), there have been reports of serious, sometimes fatal, reactions including hyperthermia, rigidity, myoclonus, autonomic instability with possible rapid fluctuations of vital signs, and mental status changes that include extreme agitation progressing to delirium and coma. These reactions have also been reported in patients who have recently discontinued that drug and have been started on an MAOI. Some cases presented with features resembling neuroleptic malignant syndrome. Therefore, it is recommended that SRIs not be used in combination with an MAOI or within 14 days of discontinuing treatment with an MAOI. Similarly, at least 14 days should be allowed after stopping an SRI before starting an MAOI.

Common Adverse Effects

CNS. Insomina, nervousness, drowsiness, fatigue, tremor, sweating, dizziness, and anxiety with fluoxetine; headache with paroxetine; dry mouth with paroxetine and sertraline; male sexual dysfunction (ejaculatory delay) with sertraline.

GI. Nausea, anorexia, diarrhea or loose stools, and constipation with paroxetine; dyspepsia with fluoxetine and sertraline.

Pregnancy

Patients should be advised to notify their physician if they become pregnant or intend to become pregnant during therapy.

Labor and Delivery

The effect of paroxetine on labor and delivery in humans is unknown.

Nursing Mothers

Patients should be advised to notify their physician if they are breast-feeding an infant. SRIs may be secreted in human milk, and caution should be exercised when an SRI is administered to a nursing woman.

Overdosage and Toxicity

No deaths were reported following the acute overdosage with paroxetine alone or in combination with other drugs and/or alcohol during premarketing clinical trials. Signs and symptoms of overdosage include nausea, vomiting, drowsiness, sinus tachycardia, and dilated pupils. There were no reports of ECG abnormalities, coma, or convulsions following overdosage with paroxetine alone. As of November 1992, there were 79 reports of nonfatal acute overdoses involving sertraline of which 28 involved sertraline alone and the remainder involved a combination of other drugs and/or alcohol with sertraline. In those cases of overdose involving only sertraline, the reported doses ranged from 500 to 6,000 mg. In a subset of 18 of these patients in whom sertraline blood levels were determined, plasma concentrations ranged from <5 to 554 ng/ml. Although there were no reports of death when sertraline was taken alone, there were 4 deaths involving overdoses of sertraline in combination with other drugs and/or alcohol. Therefore, any overdose should be treated aggressively.

Manifestations. Symptoms of overdose with sertraline alone included somnolence, nausea, tachycardia, ECG changes, anxiety, and dilated pupils.

Overdosage Management. Treatment was primarily supportive and included monitoring of and use of activated charcoal, gastric lavage, or cathartics and hydration. Establish and maintain an airway; ensure adequate oxygenation and ventilation. Activated charcoal, which may be used with sorbitol, may be as or more effective than emesis or lavage, and should be considered in treating overdose. Cardiac and vital signs monitoring is recommended along with general symptomatic and supportive measures. There are no specific antidotes for sertraline. Due to the large volume of distribution of sertraline, forced diuresis, dialysis, hemoperfusion, and exchange transfusion are unlikely to be of benefit. In managing overdosage, consider the possibility of multiple drug involvement. Treatment should consist of those general measures employed in the management of overdosage with any antidepressant. There are no specific antidotes for paroxetine. Establish and maintain an airway; ensure adequate oxygenation and ventilation. Gastric evacuation either by the induction of emesis or lavage or both should be performed. In most cases, following evacuation, 20 to 30 grams of activated charcoal may be administered every 4 to 6 hours during the first 24 to 48 hours after ingestion. An ECG should be taken and monitoring of cardiac function instituted if there is any evidence of abnormality. Supportive care with frequent monitoring of vital signs and careful observation is indicated. Due to the large volume of distribution of paroxetine, forced diuresis, dialysis, hemoperfusion, and exchange transfusion are unlikely to be of benefit.

A specific caution involves patients taking or recently having taken paroxetine who might ingest by accident or intent excessive quantities of a tricyclic antidepressant. In such a case, accumulation of the parent tricyclic and its active metabolite may increase the possibility of clinically significant sequelae and extend the time needed for close medical observation. In managing overdosage, consider the possibility of multiple-drug involvement.

FLUOXETINE

Pharmacology

Fluoxetine is chemically unrelated to tricyclic, tetracyclic, or other available antidepressants. It is believed to exert its antidepressant effects by inhibition of neuronal uptake of serotonin. In the usual clinical doses it does not block reuptake of norepinephrine.

Pharmacokinetics

Absorption. Fluoxetine is absorbed equally whether food is present or absent. Peak serum levels are achieved approximately 6 to 8 hours after ingestion.

Distribution. Approximately 95% of fluoxetine is bound to serum proteins.

Elimination. Fluoxetine is demethylated to norfluoxetine, an active metabolite. This is further metabolized by the liver to inactive compounds. Fluoxetine has an elimination half-life of 2 to 3 days and its active metabolite norfluoxetine has an elimination half-life of 7 to 9 days. When patients are maintained on a fixed dose, steady-state plasma concentrations are achieved only after several weeks of continual administration of the drug. These long elimination half-lives produce active drug in the serum for several weeks after discontinuation of administration. In liver disease such as cirrhosis, the mean elimination half-life can more than double. For this reason fluoxetine should be used with caution in such patients. Furthermore, accumulation of fluoxetine and its metabolites may occur in patients with impaired renal function.

Uses

Fluoxetine is an antidepressant drug. However, its antidepressant action has not been fully evaluated in hospitalized depressed patients. Likewise its efficacy for use longer than 5 to 6 weeks has not been systematically evaluated in controlled trials. For both of these populations, physicians should periodically reexamine patients to assess both the benefit and continued indication for the drug. High dosages of fluoxetine (of approximately 80 mg/day) have also been shown to be effective in the treatment of obsessive-compulsive disorder.

Cautions

Adverse Effects. Anxiety and insomnia occur in approximately 10% to 15% of patients receiving fluoxetine. Rarely, these symptoms may be severe enough to warrant discontinuation of the drug. Weight loss, associated with a reduction in appetite, also may occur with fluoxetine. In approximately 10% of patients the loss will be greater than 5% of body weight. Fluoxetine shares some risks associated with all antidepressants, including the possibility of switching into hypomania or mania, or the development of seizures. Both of these problems occur about as commonly with TCAs as they do with fluoxetine. Fluoxetine may impair concentration and psychomotor skills. For this reason patients should be cautioned about engaging in hazardous activities, including operating machinery and driving an automobile while under the influence of fluoxetine.

Common reasons for the discontinuation of fluoxetine include nervousness, anxiety, insomnia, nausea, and, in some cases, dizziness or tremor.

Cardiovascular effects, including conduction disturbances, are rare. Likewise, endocrinologic and hematopoietic system side effects are infrequent. Fluoxetine may produce abnormal and vivid dreams.

Precautions and Contraindications

A long elimination half-life of fluoxetine (2–3 days) and its major active metabolite (7–9 days) has practical clinical implications. Changes in dose will not be fully reflected in the plasma for several weeks. Therefore conventional strategies for dose titration and drug withdrawal need modification with this point in mind. Likewise, caution should be used in those patients with systemic illness which could affect the metabolism of fluoxetine.

The manufacturer recommends avoiding the combined use of MAOIs and fluoxetine. The manufacturer further recommends that at least 14 days elapse between discontinuation of an MAOI and initiation of fluoxetine. Because of the long half-life of fluoxetine and its active metabolites, the manufacturer also recommends that at least 5 weeks elapse between the discontinuation of fluoxetine and the initiation of an MAOI.

The manufacturer reports that approximately 4% of patients developed a rash during premarketing evaluation. The rash is associated in some cases with fever, leukocytosis, arthralgias, edema, respiratory distress, lymphadenopathy, proteinuria, and a mild transaminase elevation. Most patients improved with the discontinuation of fluoxetine. Some patients required adjunctive treatment with antihistamines or steroids. All patients who experienced the rash and accompanying events were reported to have recovered completely.

Toxicity

Prominent symptoms of overdose include nausea and vomiting, agitation, restlessness, hypomania, and general CNS excitation. Patients may experience grand mal seizures. These seizures may be arrested by the administration of a benzodiazepine such as diazepam. In dogs who have received overdoses of fluoxetine there has been no alteration in the ECG. In particular, there has not been prolongation of the PR, QRS, or QT intervals. However, the manufacturer does recommend monitoring the ECG in cases of human overdose. Early in the course of an overdose, activated charcoal may be effective. General supportive measures should be undertaken with concurrent cardiac and vital signs monitoring.

Drug Interactions

The concomitant use of tryptophan may produce a syndrome characterized by agitation, restlessness, myoclonus, and GI distress. Drugs which are highly protein-bound may be displaced by fluoxetine. This may cause a shift in plasma concentrations and result in an adverse effect. When administered with TCAs, elevated levels of tricyclic drugs may result. Enhanced sedative effects of serotonergic antidepressants have been reported. According to the manufacturer's recommendation the combined use of an MAOI and fluoxetine is contraindicated; otherwise at least 14 days should elapse between discontinuation of an MAOI and initiation of fluoxetine, and again because of the long half-lives of fluoxetine and its active metabolite, at least 5 weeks should elapse between discontinuing it and initiating an MAOI; otherwise, a hazardous and fatal reaction could occur. Recent case reports document a possible synergistic reaction between fluoxetine and lithium.

The concurrent administration of tryptophan may produce a syndrome characterized by agitation, restlessness, and GI distress. Drugs which are highly protein-bound may be displaced by fluoxetine. This may cause a shift in plasma concentration and result in an adverse effect.

Dosage and Administration

Dosage. A dose of 20 mg/day is the usual way to initiate treatment. This may be increased after several weeks if no clinical improvement is observed. Doses above 20 mg are usually administered in divided doses with the initial dose in the morning and the second dose at noon. The antidepressant effect may require 4 weeks or longer. In patients with obsessive-compulsive disorder, dosages ranging from 80 to 120 mg have been employed. Dosage is gradually titrated upward in 20-mg increments as tolerated.

Patients with renal or hepatic disease should receive less frequent and lower dosages.

Administration. Fluoxetine is administered orally.

Preparations

Fluoxetine (*Prozac*)
Oral capsules
20 mg

FLUVOXAMINE

Pharmacology

Fluvoxamine is a serotonin reuptake inhibitor (SRI) chemically unrelated to other SRIs, tricyclics, or other available antidepressants. It may exert its antiobsessional and antidepressant effects by inhibition of neuronal uptake of serotonin. In the usual clinical doses, it does not block reuptake of norepinephrine. In vitro, it has little affinity for histaminergic, adrenergic, muscarinic, or dopaminergic receptors.

Pharmacokinetics

Absorption. The bioavailability of fluvoxamine is approximately 50% and is not affected by food.

Distribution. Approximately 80% of fluvoxamine is bound to serum proteins.

Elimination. Fluvoxamine is primarily metabolized by the liver. Its metabolites only minimally inhibit serotonin reuptake. Fluvoxamine has an elimination half-life of 16 hours. In patients with liver disease, the clearance is reduced by approximately 30%. In the elderly, mean plasma concentrations are almost 40% higher than in younger patients on the same dose. Thus, fluvoxamine should be used with caution in patients with hepatic disease and in the elderly. Renal dysfunction does not appear to reduce clearance.

Uses

Fluvoxamine is approved in the United States for treatment of obsessive-compulsive disorder (OCD). Its efficacy for longer than 10 weeks has not been evaluated in controlled trials. Many placebo-controlled and double-blind studies have also established it as an effective antidepressant.

Cautions

See information under the general statement for SRIs.

Adverse Effects. In treatment studies, 22% of patients dropped out because of adverse effects. Of those patients, 9% experienced nausea, 4% insomnia, 4% somnolence, and 3% headache.

Fluvoxamine, like all antidepressants, may induce hypomania or mania (approximately 1% of patients).

Fluvoxamine produces electrolytic, hematologic, urinary, or cardiovascular reactions no more frequently than a placebo.

Precautions and Contraindications

Administration of fluvoxamine with terfenadine or astemizole is contraindicated (see *Drug Interactions).*

Since the combination of other SRIs with monoamine oxidase inhibitors (MAOI) can produce autonomic instability, hyperthermia, myoclonus, and fatalities, fluvoxamine should not be used less than 14 days before or after the administration of an MAOI (see the *General Statement* on SRIs).

Caution should be used in prescribing fluvoxamine to geriatric patients and to patients with hepatic illness.

Toxicity

Three hundred forty-five cases of accidental or deliberate overdose with fluvoxamine have been reported. Nineteen of these (5%) died. Two patients took fluvoxamine alone while the rest took fluvoxamine with other drugs. Eighty-seven percent of the overdose victims recovered completely. Frequent symptoms of overdose include somnolence, vomiting, diarrhea, and agitation. To manage the overdose patient, general supportive measures should be undertaken including concurrent cardiac and vital signs monitoring. Please see the *General Statement* on SRIs.

Drug Interactions

Fluvoxamine appears to inhibit the cytochrome P450 IA2, IIC9, and IIIA4 isoenzymes. Because theophylline, propranolol, warfarin, alprazolam, terfenadine, and astemizole are metabolized by these isoenzymes, their use with fluvoxamine must be undertaken with some caution. Since warfarin, theophylline, and phenytoin have narrow therapeutic ratios, plasma levels of these drugs may be advisable during concomitant treatment with fluvoxamine. Astemizole and terfenadine are contraindicated because elevated levels of these drugs have been linked to QT prolongation, torsades de pointes, and fatalities.

Dosage

Fluvoxamine is usually started at 50 mg in a single daily dose. The controlled trials establishing its efficacy for OCD used doses of 100–300 mg per day. Thus, the dose should be increased every 4–7 days in 50-mg increments to a final dose of 100–300 mg/day. Doses above 100 mg are usually administered in divided doses. Elderly patients or patients with hepatic disease should receive less frequent and lower doses. Antidepressant doses are similar to those for OCD.

Administration. Fluvoxamine is administered orally.

Preparations

Fluvoxamine (*Luvox*)
  Oral tablets
    50 mg, 100 mg

NEFAZODONE

Pharmacology

Nefazodone is a phenylpiperazine compound and structural analogue of trazodone. It is also similar in pharmacology to trazodone but associated with less sedation. It causes postsynaptic serotonin 2A (5HT-2A) antagonism and presynaptic serotonergic reuptake inhibition. It is thought that these actions lead to postsynaptic serotonin receptor down regulation while enhancing 5HT-2A activity. The latter occurs because 5HT-2A effects include inhibition of 5HT-1A receptor activity.

Nefazodone has no dopaminergic activity and no inhibitory effect on monoamine oxidase. It has low anticholinergic activity. There is some noradrenergic reuptake inhibition that is lost with chronic administration. Compared to trazodone, there is much less alpha-adrenergic blockade and, therefore, less orthostatic hypotension and less risk of priapism. Compared to trazodone, nefazodone also has less antihistaminic activity and, therefore, causes less sedation and weight gain. Nefazodone is the only antidepressant that does not suppress rapid eye movement (REM) during sleep.

Pharmacokinetics

Absorption. Nefazodone is almost completely absorbed after oral administration, but is then subject to extensive first-pass metabolism, which limits the absolute bioavailability to approximately 20%.

Food may delay and decrease absorption, but this does not appear to be clinically significant.

Distribution. Peak plasma levels are obtained in 1–2 hours. There is no evidence of a relationship between plasma concentrations and therapeutic effect. Nefazodone is highly (greater than 99%) protein bound; therefore, nefazodone may, in theory, displace and increase the free concentrations of other highly protein-bound drugs.

Elimination. Nefazodone undergoes extensive hepatic hydroxylation and dealkylation to form three major metabolites: hydroxynefazodone (OH-nefazodone), triazoledione (desethyl hydroxynefazodone), and m-chlorophenylpiperazine (mCPP).

OH-nefazodone has pharmacologic activity that is very similar to nefazodone. Triazoledione is one-seventh as potent as nefazodone at the SHT-2A receptors with no effect on serotonin reuptake. The mCPP metabolite, which is a minor metabolite, has weak (and probably clinically insignificant) agonist effects at the 5HT-lA, 1C, and 5HT-3 receptors. The elimination half-life of nefazodone ranges from 2–8 hours. The average half-life of total nefazodone (including metabolites) is 11–24 hours. Steady state is achieved in about 5 days. Nefazodone is eliminated primarily, as its metabolites, in both urine and feces. Clearance of nefazodone may decrease in elderly patients and those with hepatic impairment.

Uses

The only FDA-approved use of nefazodone is for the treatment of depression. It may have particular efficacy with symptoms of anxiety associated with depression. Several weeks of treatment may be required to achieve full antidepressant effect. Nefazodone may also have some use in the treatment of symptom-associated premenstrual syndromes.

Cautions

Adverse Effects. Overall, in clinical trials nefazodone was better tolerated than imipramine and appears to be relatively free of the restlessness and insomnia that are often associated with treatment with the selective serotonin reuptake inhibitors (SSRIs). Nefazodone caused somnolence, dry mouth, and nausea in 22%–25% of patients. Other side effects with low-to-moderate incidence include dizziness, constipation, asthenia, light-headedness, and blurred vision. There has been no significant incidence of weight change or sexual dysfunction. In the clinical trials, 16% of the patients discontinued treatment because of adverse effects (compared with 20% on TCAs and 10% on placebo). Although nefazodone does not seem to pose a significant risk for adverse cardiovascular effects, it has not been studied in patients with preexisting cardiac disease.

Precautions and Contraindications

There is a low risk of postural hypotension. Nefazodone should be used with caution in patients with known cardiovascular or cerebrovascular disease that could be exacerbated by hypotension. Terfenadine and astemizole are contraindicated with nefazodone. Concomitant treatment with MAOIs is also contraindicated.

Toxicity

Overdose is expected to be associated with low toxicity. Overdoses of 1,000–11,000 mg have resulted in nausea, vomiting, and somnolence. There is one report of seizures following ingestion of 2,000–3,000 mg of nefazodone together with methocarbamol and alcohol. There are no reports of fatal overdoses.

Drug Interactions

Nefazodone is highly protein bound; therefore, caution is warranted when coadministering with other highly protein-bound drugs, even though in vitro testing with several such drugs failed to show an interaction. Nefazodone is a potent inhibitor of the cytochrome P450-IIIA4 isoenzyme and a weak inhibitor of the IID6 isoenzyme. Therefore, drugs that rely on these enzymes for their metabolism may have increased levels and adverse effects when administered with nefazodone. Such drugs include terfenadine and astemizole, which are contraindicated with nefazodone, and triazolam and alprazolam, which require dose reductions of 75% and 50%, respectively. Other such drugs include nifedipine, cocaine, cyclosporine, testosterone, risperidone, haloperidol, clozapine, TCAs, thioridazine, perphenazine, venlafaxine, propranolol, codeine, and paroxetine; dose reductions of these drugs may be necessary. Therapeutic doses of nefazodone may result in additive cognitive and psychomotor impairment when combined with alcohol. Careful monitoring of digoxin levels are recommended when using nefazodone with other drugs. Nefazodone may potentiate opiate effects via a possible action on the opioid receptors.

When switching from an MAOI to nefazodone, a 2-week washout period is recommended. When switching from nefazodone to an MAO1, a 1-week washout is recommended.

Dosage and Administration Dosage

Nefazodone is effective in a dose range of 300–600 mg/day. In healthy young adults, treatment is initiated at 100-mg twice daily and titrated every 4–7 days until symptoms start resolving or until a dose of 300–600 mg/day is reached.

In healthy elderly patients or in those patients with coexisting medical problems, dosing should be initiated at 50 mg twice daily and titrated up weekly as tolerated. The 100-mg tablet is scored. In the elderly, 200–400 mg/day is the usual effective dose, but the final dose may be the same as in younger patients.

Administration. Nefazodone is administered orally.

Preparations

Nefazodone (*Serzone*)
  Oral tablets
    100, 150, 200, 250 mg

PAROXETINE HYDROCHLORIDE

Pharmacology

Paroxetine is an orally administered antidepressant with a chemical structure unrelated to other serotonin reuptake inhibitors or to tricyclic, tetracyclic, or other available antidepressant agents. It is the hydrochloride salt of a phenylpiperidine compound. The antidepressant action of paroxetine is presumed to be linked to potentiation of serotonergic activity in the central nervous system resulting from inhibition of neuronal reuptake of serotonin. Paroxetine is a potent and highly selective inhibitor of neuronal serotonin reuptake and has only very weak effects on norepinephrine and dopamine neuronal reuptake. In vitro radioligand binding studies indicate that paroxetine has little affinity for muscarinic α_1-, α_2-, β-adrenergic-, dopamine (D2)-, 5-HT1-, 5-HT2,- and histamine (H1)-receptors.

Pharmacokinetics

Absorption. Paroxetine is completely absorbed after oral dosing. Steady-state concentrations are achieved by 10 days for most subjects. At steady state, mean values of Cmax, Tmax, Cmin, and T1/12 were 61.7 ng/ml (CV 45%), 5.2 hr (CV 10%), 30.7 ng/ml (CV 67%), and 21 hr (CV 32%), respectively.

Distribution. Paroxetine distributes throughout the body, including the CNS.

Elimination. Paroxetine is extensively metabolized after oral administration. The principal metabolites are polar and conjugated products of oxidation and methylation, which are readily cleared. The metabolites have no more than 1/50 the potency of the parent compound at inhibiting serotonin uptake and are, therefore, essentially inactive. The metabolism of paroxetine is accomplished in part by cytochrome P450IID6. The role of this enzyme in paroxetine metabolism suggests potential drug-drug interactions (see *Precautions*). Approximately 93% to 95% of paroxetine is bound to plasma proteins.

Approximately 64% of a 30-mg oral solution dose of paroxetine is excreted in the urine with 2% as the parent and 62% as metabolites over a 10-day postdosing period. About 36% was excreted in the feces (probably via the bile) mostly as metabolites and less than 1% as the parent compound over the same period. Elevated plasma concentrations of paroxetine occur in subjects with renal and hepatic impairment. The mean plasma concentrations in patients with creatinine clearance below 30 ml/min was approximately 4 times greater than seen in normal volunteers. Patients with creatine clearance of 30 to 60 ml/min and patients with hepatic functional impairment had about a twofold increase in plasma concentrations (AUC, Cmax). The initial dosage should therefore be reduced in patients with severe renal or hepatic impairment, and upward titration, if necessary, should be at increased intervals (see *Dosage and Administration*).

In a multiple-dose study in the elderly at daily paroxetine doses of 20, 30, and 40 mg, Cmin concentrations were about 70% to 80% greater than the respective Cmin concentrations in nonelderly subjects. Therefore, the initial dosage in the elderly should be reduced (see *Dosage and Administration*).

Uses

Paroxetine hydrochloride is indicated for the treatment of major depressive disorders. The efficacy of paroxetine in maintaining an antidepressant response for up to 1 year has been demonstrated in a placebo-controlled trial. Nevertheless, the physician who uses paroxetine for extended periods should periodically reevaluate its long-term effectiveness.

Cautions

Adverse Effects. Of patients given this drug, 21% discontinued treatment due to an adverse event. The most commonly observed adverse events (incidence of 5% or greater) were asthenia, sweating, nausea, decreased appetite, somnolence, dizziness, insomnia, tremor, nervousness, ejaculatory disturbance, and other male genital disorders. In a fixed-dose study comparing adverse event rates of paroxetine given at 10, 20, 30, and 40 mg/day with a placebo revealed a clear dose dependency for some of the more common adverse events associated with paroxetine use. Over a 4- to 6-week period, there was evidence of adaptation to some adverse events with continued therapy (e.g., nausea and dizziness), but less to other effects (e.g., dry mouth, somnolence, and asthenia).

Drug Interactions

MAOIs. There is a potential for interaction with monoamine oxidase inhibitors. In patients receiving serotonin reuptake drugs in combination with a monoamine oxidase inhibitor (MAOI), there have been reports of serious, sometimes fatal, reactions, including hyperthermia, rigidity, myoclonus, autonomic instability with possible rapid fluctuations of vital signs, and mental status changes that include extreme agitation progressing to delirium and coma. These reactions have also been reported in patients who have recently discontinued that drug and have started on a MAOI. Some cases presented with features resembling neuroleptic malignant syndrome. It is recommended that paroxetine not be used in combination with a MAOI or within 14 days of discontinuing treatment with a MAOI. At least 2 weeks should be allowed after stopping paroxetine before starting a MAOI. At least 14 days should elapse between discontinuation of a MAOI and initiation of paroxetine therapy. Similarly, at least 14 days should be allowed after stopping paroxetine before starting a MAOI.

Dosage and Administration

Paroxetine should be administered as a single daily dose, usually in the morning. The recommended initial dose is 20 mg/day. Patients were dosed in a range of 20 to 50 mg/day in the clinical trials demonstrating the antidepressant effectiveness of paroxetine. As with all antidepressants, the full antidepressant effect may be delayed. Some patients not responding to a 20–mg dose may benefit from dose increases (in 10–mg/day increments) up to a maximum of 50 mg/day. Dose changes should occur at intervals of at least 1 week.

The recommended initial dose is 10 mg/day for elderly patients, debilitated patients, and/or patients with severe renal or hepatic impairment. Increases may be made if indicated. Dosage should not exceed 40 mg/day.

Usage in Children. Safety and effectiveness in children have not been established.

Geriatric Use. Pharmacokinetic studies reveal a decreased clearance in the elderly. A lower starting dose is recommended. There are no overall differences in adverse event profile between elderly and younger patients. Effectiveness is similar in younger and older patients.

It is generally agreed that acute episodes of depression require several months of sustained pharmacologic therapy. Whether the dose of an antidepressant needed to induce remission is identical to the dose needed to maintain and/or sustain euthymia is unknown. Systemic evaluation of the efficacy of paroxetine has shown that efficacy is maintained for periods up to 1 year with doses that averaged about 30 mg.

Preparations

Paroxetine is supplied as follows:

20 mg
30 mg
Brand names: *Aropax; Paxil; Seroxat*

SERTRALINE HYDROCHLORIDE

Sertraline is an antidepressant for oral administration. It is chemically unrelated to tricyclic, tetracyclic, or other available antidepressant agents. Sertraline hydrochloride is a white crystalline powder that is slightly soluble in water and isopropyl alcohol and sparingly soluble in ethanol.

Uses

Sertraline is indicated for the treatment of major depression. However, the effectiveness of sertraline in long-term use (for more than 16 weeks) has not been systematically evaluated in controlled trials. Therefore, the physician who elects to use sertraline for extended periods should periodically reevaluate the long-term usefulness of the drug for the individual patient.

Adverse Effects

Commonly Observed. The most commonly observed adverse events associated with the use of sertraline and not seen at an equivalent incidence among placebo-treated patients were gastrointestinal complaints, including nausea, diarrhea/loose stools, and dyspepsia; tremor; dizziness; insomnia; somnolence; increased sweating; dry mouth; and male sexual dysfunction (primarily ejaculatory delay).

Associated with Discontinuation of Treatment. Fifteen percent of subjects who received sertraline in premarketing clinical trials discontinued treatment due to an adverse event. The more common events associated with discontinuation included agitation, insomnia, male sexual dysfunction (primarily ejaculatory delay), somnolence, dizziness, headache, tremor, anorexia, diarrhea/loose stools, nausea, and fatigue.

Precautions and Contraindications

See the General Statement on SRIs.

Drug Interactions

See the General Statement on SRIs.

Dosage and Administration

Dosage. Sertraline treatment should be initiated with a dose of 50 mg once daily. While a relationship between dose and antidepressant effect has not been established, patients were dosed in a range of 50–200 mg/day in the clinical trials to demonstrate the antidepressant effectiveness of sertraline. Consequently, patients not responding to a 50-mg dose may benefit from dose increases up to a maximum of 200 mg/day. Given the 24-hour elimination half-life of sertraline, dose changes should not occur at intervals of less than 1 week. As indicated under Precautions, a lower or less frequent dosage should be used in patients with hepatic impairment. In addition, particular care should be used in patients with hepatic and/or renal impairment.

Administration. Sertraline should be administered once daily, either in the morning or evening.

Safety and effectiveness in children have not been established.

Efficacy and the pattern of adverse reactions in the elderly were similar to that in younger patients.

There is evidence to suggest that depressed patients responding during an initial 8-week treatment phase will continue to benefit during an additional 8 weeks of treatment. While there are insufficient data regarding any benefits from treatment beyond 16 weeks, it is generally agreed that acute episodes of depression require several months or longer of sustained pharmacologic therapy.

Preparations

50-mg tablet
100-mg tablet
Lustral; Zoloft

VENLAFAXINE

Pharmacology

Venlafaxine is a phenethylamine compound that is structurally unrelated to other available antidepressant agents. Venlafaxine strongly inhibits the reuptake of both norepinephrine (NE) and serotonin (5HT). Venlafaxine has no significant effect on muscarinic, histaminergic, or adrenergic receptors. The drug is a weak inhibitor of dopamine reuptake.

Venlafaxine exists as a racemic mixture of "R" and "S" enantiomers. Both enantiomers, as well as the major metabolite O-desmethyl-venlafaxine, have antidepressant activity.

Pharmacokinetics

Absorption. Venlafaxine is well absorbed following oral administration, then undergoes extensive first-pass metabolism. Food does not significantly affect the extent of absorption.

Distribution. Venlafaxine, and its active metabolite O-desmethylvenlafaxine (ODV), have low protein bindings—in the range of 27% and 30%, respectively. This is in contrast with the serotonin reuptake inhibitors (SRIs), which are all highly protein bound (>90%). Venlafaxine and ODV reach steady-state plasma concentrations within 72 hours.

Elimination. Venlafaxine undergoes extensive hepatic metabolism. The two minor metabolites, N-desmethylvenlafaxine and N,O-didesmethylvenlafaxine, are inactive; 56% of the drug is converted to its active metabolite, O-desmethylvenlafaxaine. The primary route of excretion of the drug and its metabolites is via the kidneys. The mean elimination half-life of venlafaxine is 5 hours, and that of ODV is approximately 11 hours.

There is a small reduction in steady-state clearance of venlafaxine in the elderly; however, there is no need to adjust dosing based on age. There is significant impact on clearance and elimination in patients with renal or hepatic impairments. Dosing adjustments are necessary for these patients (see section on *Dosage and Administration*).

Uses

Treatment with venlafaxine is indicated for major depression. Studies of the long-term effectiveness of venlafaxine have not been completed. There is some initial evidence, from animal studies, that the onset of action of venlafaxine may be slightly earlier than seen with other antidepressants.

Cautions

Adverse Effects. The most common adverse effects associated with venlafaxine treatment compared with placebo include nausea, dry mouth, dizziness, constipation, nervousness, sweating, asthenia, abnormal ejaculation or orgasm, and anorexia. Problems with nausea, somnolence, and dizziness decrease after the first few weeks of treatment. This is particularly true for nausea, which occurred in 29% of trial patients during the first week of treatment but decreased to 6% by the fifth week. The incidence of nausea appears to be related more to the amount of the initial dose and of the increments during titration, rather than the total daily dose.

Increases in diastolic blood pressure (of about 7 mm Hg) occur in >5% of patients who are taking more than 200 mg/day. Analysis of EKGs during venlafaxine trials revealed a mean increase in heart rate of 4 beats per minute, but no evidence of disturbance in intracardiac conduction. Mean increases of serum cholesterol of 3 mg/dL were noted among venlafaxine-treated patients. In the clinical trials, 19% of the patients stopped treatment because of adverse effects compared with 20% of patients treated with tricyclic antidepressants and 6% of placebo-treated patients.

Weight gain is not a problem with venlafaxine. In fact, a dose-dependent weight loss was reported in 11% of patients.

Seizures were reported in 0.26% of trial patients. Venlafaxine should be used with caution in patients with a history of seizures and should be discontinued in any patients who develop seizures.

Upon discontinuation of treatment with venlafaxine, the following symptoms occurred at an incidence of at least 5%: asthenia, dizziness, headache, insomnia, nausea, and nervousness. It is recommended that when discontinuing treatment, the dosage be tapered gradually.

Precautions and Contraindications

There is no contraindication to venlafaxine use in patients with hypertension; however, regular monitoring of blood pressure is recommended for all patients being treated with venlafaxine. Venlafaxine dosage may need to be reduced or discontinued for patients with sustained increases in blood pressure.

Concomitant treatment with venlafaxine and monoamine oxidase inhibitors (MAOIs) is contraindicated.

Venlafaxine, like all antidepressants, should be used cautiously in patients with a history of mania.

Toxicity

During the clinical trials, there were 14 reports of overdose with venlafaxine, with the highest amount ingested being 8.75 gm. Somnolence was the most common symptom; one patient had 2 generalized convulsions and a 25% prolongation of QTc; mild sinus tachycardia was reported in 2 patients; most patients reported no symptoms.

Drug Interactions

Venlafaxine has low protein binding; therefore, it should not increase the free concentrations of drugs that are highly protein bound. Venlafaxine is metabolized by the cytochrome P450-II6 isoenzyme; therefore, there is the possibility of interaction with drugs that inhibit the activity of this isoenzyme. The pharmacokinetic profiles of venlafaxine and lithium, diazepam, or ethanol were not significantly altered when venlafaxine was paired with one of these drugs. Nor did treatment with venlafaxine impact on the psychomotor or psychometric effects induced by diazepam or alcohol. Cimetidine does inhibit the first-pass metabolism of venlafaxine. Although no dose adjustment is required, this combination should be used with caution in elderly patients or patients with hepatic dysfunction.

When switching from an MAOI to venlafaxine, a 2-week washout period is recommended. When switching from venlafaxine to an MAOI, a 1-week washout is recommended.

Dosage and Administration

Dosage. Venlafaxine appears to be effective within a range of 75–375 mg/day. There is some suggestion of a dose response relationship in the range of 75–225 mg/day. Treatment should be initiated at 75 mg/day, in two or three divided doses, and taken with food. The dosage may be increased in increments of up to 75 mg/day at intervals of no less than 4 days. The maximum recommended dose is 375 mg/day. Doses greater than 225 mg/day are usually not needed for outpatient treatment of moderate depression.

For patients with mild-to-moderate renal impairment (glomerular filtration rates of 10–70 ml/min), the venlafaxine dose should be reduced by 25%. For patients undergoing hemodialysis, the dose should be reduced by 50% and administered 4 hours after the completion of dialysis. For patients with moderate hepatic impairment, the dosage should be reduced by 50%. Additional dosage reductions may be appropriate for some patients with renal or hepatic impairment.

No dosage adjustment is required for the treatment of elderly patients; however, careful monitoring while titrating the dose is warranted.

If a patient has been treated with venlafaxine for 1 week or more, it is recommended that the dose be tapered prior to discontinuation of treatment. This tapering should be done gradually over a 2-week period for those patients that have been treated for 6 or more weeks.

Administration. Venlafaxine is administered orally.

Preparations

Venlafaxine (*Effexor*)

Oral tablets

25, 37.5, 50, 75, and 100 mg

ANTIMANIC AGENTS 3

CARBAMAZEPINE

Pharmacology

The efficacy of carbamazepine (CBZ) in the acute and maintenance treatment of bipolar disorder is well established. Its mechanism of action is unknown in these conditions. The drug is known to have anticholinergic, antidepressant, sedative and antiarrhythmic properties. It is structurally related to the tricyclic antidepressants.

Pharmacokinetics

CBZ is well absorbed from the gastrointestinal (GI) tract. Up to 4 days may be required to achieve steady-state plasma levels. While therapeutic plasma levels have been determined for the control of epilepsy these may not apply for the control of mood disorders. The drug is widely distributed in all body tissues, including cerebrospinal fluid (CSF), brain, and of importance for the nursing mother, breast milk. It also crosses the placenta.

Elimination. Half-life averages 25 to 65 hours. Its wide variability is in part due to the fact that CBZ can induce its own metabolism by stimulating oxidation via microsomal enzymes in the liver. CBZ and its metabolites are excreted in the urine.

Uses

CBZ is effective in the treatment of acute mania and bipolar prophylaxis. During acute mania it may be used alone or with adjunctive neuroleptics. During maintenance treatment it may also be used with adjunctive depressants.

Cautions

Hematologic Effects. Hematologic consequences of carbamazepine administration include leukopenia, agranulocytosis, eosinophilia, leukocytosis, thrombocytopenia, and pancytopenia. Most commonly these are minor hematologic changes which may be transient or persistent. However, death from aplastic anemia has occurred on rare occasions with carbamazepine administration. The risk for developing aplastic anemia or agranulocytosis is five to eight times greater in patients receiving CBZ than in the general population. In general, these problems first manifest as minor hematologic changes and then progress to agranulocytosis or aplastic anemia. However, this transition occurs in only a small number of patients who have the initial minor hematologic changes described above. For this reason, however, most clinicians will obtain a baseline complete blood count (CBC) prior to the initiation of CBZ and follow the patient with periodic reexaminations.

Cardiovascular Effects. Cardiovascular effects have included hypotension, syncope, arrhythmias, atrioventricular (AV) block, and exacerbation of congestive heart failure.

Hepatic Effects. Administration of CBZ has been associated with abnormal increases in liver function tests and jaundice.

Genitourinary Effects. Generally, these are uncommon, but may include an increase in urinary frequency and urinary retention, in particular in elderly males; azotemia; and renal failure.

Nervous System Effects. A variety of adverse consequences can occur with CBZ administration. These may include ataxia, impaired coordination, confusion, drowsiness, dizziness, nystagmus, blurred vision, and headache.

GI Effects. CBZ may produce vomiting, nausea, abdominal pain, diarrhea, constipation, a reduction in appetite, and dry mouth.

Dermatologic Effects. CBZ may produce erythematous or pruritic rashes and urticaria. Less commonly there may be photosensitivity reactions and in extremely rare situations toxic epidermal necrolysis and exfoliative dermatitis.

Precautions and Contraindications

Because of the side effects associated with carbamazepine it should only be prescribed to patients who have cardiac, hepatic, or renal disease, or a history of adverse hematologic reaction to other drugs, after a careful assessment of the benefit-to-risk ratio. Patients should be alerted to the clinical signs of hematologic toxicity. They should be cautioned that fever, infection, sore throat, easy bruising, mouth ulcers, and petechial or purpuric hemorrhage should be promptly reported to their physician. Likewise, the physician should obtain a baseline CBC along with a platelet determination and follow these as clinically indicated. In particular, caution should be exercised in the administration of this drug to patients who have a history of aplastic anemia or are receiving other drugs of a myelotoxic nature.

CBZ should be discontinued if any evidence of significant bone marrow depression develops. When significant bone marrow depression arises, daily CBC, platelet, and reticulocyte counts should be performed along with bone marrow aspiration at the initial consultation.

Fully developed aplastic anemia requires intensive treatment and monitoring and special consultation. Patients should be cautioned about engaging in activities which require physical coordination or mental alertness. Because carbamazepine is a tricyclic and structurally related to other tricyclic antidepressants, the drug may cause confusion in the elderly and activate affective disorders. Furthermore, because of its mild anticholinergic activity, patients with increased intraocular pressure should be closely monitored during CBZ therapy.

Pediatric Precautions. The efficacy and safety of carbamazepine administration in children younger than 6 years has not been established.

Pregnancy, Fertility, and Lactation. The safety of CBZ administration during pregnancy has not been established. There are reports of an increased incidence of birth defects in pregnant women receiving carbamazepine. However, a causative relationship between the drug and possible birth defects has not been established. Likewise, the safe use of CBZ during breast-feeding has not been established. Similar cautions should apply and the drug should only be administered when the patient agrees to discontinue nursing.

Acute Toxicity

Manifestations. Overdosage produces ataxia, drowsiness, and dizziness which may progress to stupor, nausea, vomiting, agitation, disorientation, tremor, and abnormal reflexes. There may be mydriasis, nystagmus, flushing, and urinary retention. There may be fluctuations in blood pressure, and coma may ultimately develop. There may be an increase or a decrease in the white count and acetone urea. Treatment includes the induction of emesis or gastric lavage. In general, supportive treatment should be provided along with careful monitoring of the electrocardiogram (ECG) for cardiac arrhythmias.

Drug Interactions With Carbamazepine

Lithium, Haloperidol. CBZ may enhance the antimanic effect of lithium in treatment-refractory patients. Combined lithium-CBZ treatment may enhance a possible neurotoxic interaction despite therapeutic plasma levels of both drugs. Risk factors for developing neurotoxicity from this combination may include a history of lithium neurotoxicity or the presence of concurrent medical or neurologic illness. It is advisable that the clinician remain alert for signs of neurotoxicity, including ataxia, tremors, muscle fasciculations, hyperreflexia, and nystagmus, even in the absence of elevated plasma concentrations of either drug. Data are conflicting concerning the effect of coadministration of CBZ and haloperidol. Several reports have demonstrated CBZ to significantly lower plasma haloperidol levels, while one report found no effect and another report showed decreased blood levels of both drugs.

Phenytoin/Phenobarbital/Primidone. The plasma levels of CBZ were significantly decreased in patients receiving CBZ plus phenytoin with or without phenobarbital, and CBZ plus primidone compared to CBZ alone. The effect of CBZ on phenytoin is more variable. Increased serum phenytoin, decreased serum phenytoin, and no change in serum phenytoin have all been reported. These differences among various reports might be accounted for by variations in CBZ and phenytoin doses, duration of therapy, variation in the sample sizes, and types of study populations, or other factors.

Calcium Channel Blockers. The calcium channel blockers verapamil and diltiazem may inhibit hepatic metabolism of CBZ, thereby increasing its plasma concentration. Neurotoxicity with dizziness, nausea, ataxia, diplopia, and mental slowing has been reported to occur with the combined use of CBZ plus verapamil or CBZ plus diltiazem but has not been reported to occur with nifedipine.

Antibacterials. Administration of standard doses of erythromycin along with CBZ may produce a toxic syndrome marked by somnolence, lethargy, dizziness, diplopia, ataxia, nausea, and nystagmus. This occurs by a reduction in serum clearance of CBZ which develops because of the inhibition of hepatic metabolism. Triacetyloleandomycin (TAO, troleandomycin) may elevate CBZ plasma levels during coadministration through the inhibition of hepatic metabolism of CBZ. There have been several reports of CBZ toxicity precipitated by coadministration with TAO.

Valproic Acid. See Valproic Acid in this chapter.

Miscellaneous Drugs. CBZ has been reported to induce hyponatremia in some patients. The combined use of thiazide diuretics or furosemide with CBZ may produce severe, symptomatic hyponatremia. Clinicians should be cautious with the combination of CBZ, lithium, and diuretics because of the potential for electrolyte depletion, which may further enhance the risk of lithium intoxication. Coadministration of CBZ with warfarin (Coumadin) may decrease warfarin elimination half-life and plasma levels. When CBZ is coadministered, the dose of warfarin may need to be increased to maintain a therapeutic prothrombin time. Correspondingly, the warfarin dose may need to be tailored when CBZ is discontinued. Cimetidine, isoniazid, and dextropropoxyphene may inhibit the metabolism and clearance of CBZ, leading to increased blood levels and potential toxicity of CBZ. Some reports indicate the interaction between CBZ and cimetidine is transient and time-dependent; after 7 days of coadministration there was no effect of cimetidine on CBZ levels. Studies have found no effect of cimetidine on CBZ or CBZ 10,11-epoxide levels in epileptic patients. CBZ may decrease the half-life of doxycycline by inducing hepatic microsomal enzymes. CBZ may also increase the metabolism of oral contraceptives. Because CBZ is a tricyclic, caution should be exercised when monoamine oxidase inhibitors (MAOIs) are also used. Manufacturers have recommended that at least 14 days elapse between discontinuation of MAOIs and initiation of treatment with CBZ. Data suggest that CBZ metabolism may be impaired by viloxazine (a second-generation antidepressant that has little or no epileptogenic potential). The physician prescribing viloxazine to patients on CBZ therapy must monitor for signs of CBZ toxicity and plasma CBZ levels.

The drug interactions with CBZ are summarized in Table 3–1.

Dosage and Administration

Dosage. The dosage of carbamazepine should be titrated to the individual's needs and tolerance. Initial administration should begin at a low dose and be gradually titrated upward. The oral suspension may produce higher peak serum concentrations. For this reason it should be initiated at smaller, more frequent dosages spread out over the day. Dosage is usually begun at 200 mg twice a day and increased up to 800 to 1,200 mg/day.

Administration. Carbamazepine is administered orally. It is best tolerated when administered with meals.

Preparations

Carbamazepine
- Oral suspension (*Tegretol*)
  - 100 mg/5 mL
- Tablets (*Epitol, Tegretol*)
  - 200 mg
- Tablets, chewable (*Tegretol*)
  - 100 mg

LITHIUM

Pharmacology

Lithium has no known physiologic function. Its numerous pharmacologic effects have not been fully clarified. It does compete with sodium, calcium, and magnesium at sites in the body. It also interacts with cyclic adenosine monophosphate. It inhibits adenylate cyclase and guanosine monophosphate.

Nervous System Effects. The mechanism of lithium's antidepressant and antimanic effects is unknown. The effects, however, appear to involve monoamine neurotransmitters, including indolamines such as serotonin and particularly catecholamines such as dopamine and norepinephrine.

Hematologic Effects. Lithium may produce an increase in red cell and platelet counts and a decrease in lymphocyte counts. Neutrophilia is the most frequent hematologic effect. Lithium causes an increase in neutrophili production and survival time, rather than simple demargination. The effect usually occurs within 3 to 7 days after initiation of lithium and reverses within 1 to 2 weeks after discontinuation of lithium.

Table 3–1.
Drug Interactions With Carbamazepine

Combination	Interaction	Mechanism/ Comment	Clinical Significance
Acetaminophen	↓ Therapeutic effects of acetaminophen	CBZ enhances acetaminophen hepatic metabolism	
	↑ Potential hepatotoxicity of acetaminophen	Toxicity occurs with large or chronic doses (?) of CBZ	?
Anticoagulants, oral warfarin (Coumadin)	↓ Anticoagulant effect of warfarin (↓ warfarin levels)	CBZ enhances warfarin hepatic metabolism Monitor prothrombin times after beginning or stopping CBZ therapy and adjust warfarin doses	Yes
Barbiturates (e.g., Phenobarbital), primidone (Mysoline)	↓ CBZ plasma concentrations	Barbiturate induction of CBZ hepatic metabolism (epoxidation), and ↑ CBZ clearance	?
Cimetidine (Tagamet), isoniazid (INH), propoxyphene (Darvon, Darvon-N) | Phenylbutazone effect;	↑ Blood levels and potential toxicity of CBZ, e.g., somnolence, lethargy, dizziness, blurred vision, ataxia, nausea, nystagmus	Inhibit hepatic metabolism of CBZ Most data indicate cimetidine-CBZ interaction is transient Ranitidine, antacid, or sucralfate might be an alternative Significantly increase CBZ serum levels in isoniazid-CBZ and propoxyphene-CBZ combination CBZ-isoniazid: double interaction (?) (i.e., ↑ isoniazid hepatotoxicity?)	Yes

Clonazepam	↓ Clonazepam effect	Induction of clonazepam hepatic metabolism by CBZ Transient effect?	?
Danazol (Danocrine)	↑↑ CBZ serum levels and risk of CBZ intoxication	Danazol inhibitionn of CBZ metabolic degradation	Yes
Doxycycline (Vibramycin)	↓ Serum levels of doxycycline, possibly reducing its therapeutic efficacy	CBZ may increase hepatic metabolism of doxycycline	Yes
Erythromycin, triacetyloleandomycin (TAO)	↑ CBZ serum levels and potential toxicity (rapid or delayed onset)	Inhibition of hepatic metabolism of CBZ (↓ CBZ clearance, ↑ CBZ accumulation Avoid this combination; otherwise closely monitor CBZ levels and signs of toxicity	Yes
Haloperidol	↓↓ Haloperidol serum levels	Mechanism ? Conflicting data; most reports have demonstrated CBZ to significantly lower plasma haloperidol levels	Yes
Hydantoins-phenytoin (Dilantin)	Phenytoin lowers CBZ serum concentrations Effect of CBZ on phenytoin is variable	Phenytoin may induce CBZ metabolism Mechanism of effect of CBZ on phenytoin unknown? Monitor serum concentrations of both drugs, especially when starting or stopping 1 drug	Yes

(Continued.)

Table 3–1 (cont.).

Combination	Interaction	Mechanism/ Comment	Clinical Significance
Hydrochlorothiazide, furosemide	Enhance hyponatremia	CBZ may increase synthesis/ or release of vasopressin	Yes
Isotretinoin	May ↓ CBZ effect	Unknown mechanism Single case report	?
Lithium	↑ Antimanic effect ↑ Lithium intoxication	Mechanism? ↓ Lithium renal clearance (intoxication may appear with normal levels of both	Yes
	? CBZ inhibits lithium polyuria	Antidiuretic action of CBZ Monitor signs of neurotoxicity, particularly when patients are at high risk (e.g., previous history of lithium neurotoxicity, or concurrent with medical or neurologic disorders)	
Mebendazole	↓ Mebendazole effects	Mechanism ? One case reported suggested	?
Monoamine oxidate inhibitors (MAOIs) (see Chapter 1)			
Muscle relaxants (nondepolarizing group) pancuronium (Pavulon), tubocurarine,etc.	↓ Therapeutic effects of muscle relaxants	Pancuronium and CBZ my compete for sites at neuromuscular junction demethylation and hydroxylation)	Yes

		Muscle relaxant dosage may need to be raised	
Theophyllines: aminophylline, theophylline, oxtriphylline	Theophylline and CBZ levels may be decreased	? Mechanism (mutual induction of hepatic metabolism may occur) Few case reports	?
Verapamil, diltiazem (? other calcium channel blockers)	↑ CBZ serum concentration and potential of intoxication	Inhibit hepatic metabolism of CBZ CBZ dose may need to be decreased 40%–50% when coadministered with verapamil Observe for signs of CBZ intoxication	Yes
Viloxazine	↑ CBZ serum levels and potential CBZ toxicity	Mechanism? Probably involves inhibition of metabolism of both CBZ and its active metabolite CBZ 10, 11-epoxide	Yes

Renal Effects. Lithium commonly produces polyuria. This is a mild manifestation of nephrogenic diabetes insipidus. Because of lithium's capability to reduce renal concentrating ability, this occurs via a reduction in water reabsorption and an increase in sodium excretion. The reduction in renal concentrating ability may persist in approximately 25% of patients on long-term lithium treatment. In most cases, it reverses with drug discontinuation. The diabetes insipidus associated with lithium can be treated by the use of triamterene, amiloride, or thiazide diuretics.

Endocrine Effects. Lithium produces hypothyroidism. There is an inhibition of release of both thyroxine (T_4) and triiodothyronine (T_3). This results in an increase in serum thyrotropin. Lithium may also produce hypoparathyroidism.

Cardiac Effects. T wave depression and inversion may occur. The depression occurs frequently. Inversion is rarely seen. Arrhythmias are rare.

Pharmacokinetics

Absorption. Lithium is easily absorbed from the GI tract. Lithium citrate solutions are 100% absorbed. Lithium carbonate capsules and tablets are likewise 100% absorbed. Extended-release lithium carbonate tablets are 60% to 90% absorbed. This absorption peaks anywhere between 30 minutes and 3 hours after administration and is completed within 1 to 6 hours after administration for lithium carbonate tablets and capsules. Extended-release preparations have a prolonged period of absorption. Their absorption is delayed and usually occurs 4 to 12 hours after administration. Steady-state serum concentrations of lithium are measured approximately 12 hours after the last dose. It is at this time that fluctuations in serum levels are at their lowest. Twelve-hour serum levels should be in the range of 0.6 to 1.2 mEq/L for a therapeutic effect. Higher levels, up to 1.5 mEq/L, are occasionally required for acute antimanic treatment. The onset of lithium's effects begins within 5 to 7 days after administration. The full effect requires 14 to 21 days.

Distribution. Lithium is distributed into both extracellular fluid and tissues. Lithium is found in breast milk at concentrations from one-third to one-half of those found in serum. It also crosses the placenta in concentrations equal to those in the maternal circulation.

Elimination. Lithium has a half-life of approximately 1 day. In the elderly and in those with impaired renal function, the half-life is 36 hours or longer. Lithium is excreted via the kidneys. In general, young patients and pregnant women have higher lithium renal clearances; clearances are lower in the geriatric population. Lithium is readily removed by hemodialysis. This is sometimes useful in overdose situations. Hemodialysis is more effective than peritoneal dialysis.

Uses

Acute Mania. Lithium is effective in the treatment of the acute manic phase of bipolar disorder and mixed bipolar states. In general 2 to 3 weeks are required for lithium to effectively control a manic or hypomanic episode. It is most effective in milder forms of mania and hypomania. During the acute period of mania or hypomania and prior to the onset of lithium's therapeutic actions, adjunctive neuroleptics or high-potency benzodiazepines are often used for acute control. These agents are particularly helpful in treating the increased psychomotor activity associated with mania. The benzodiazepines are tapered and discontinued as the clinical impact of lithium occurs.

Major Depression. Lithium is an effective antidepressant. It is more effective in patients with bipolar depression than in those with unipolar major depression. The antidepressant efficacy of lithium is approximately similar to that of the tricyclic antidepressants. In general, however, the use of lithium as an antidepressant is a second-line approach used in those who have not adequately responded to other more conventional antidepressant treatments. Lithium does appear to be effective in preventing depressive relapse.

Prophylaxis of Bipolar Disorder. Lithium effectively prevents the recurrence of bipolar manic and depressive episodes in approximately 75% of manic patients. While the decision to implement long-term lithium maintenance treatment in a bipolar patient must be made in light of the prior history, most clinicians recommend long-term lithium use in patients who have had two or more episodes of manic-depressive disease or who have had one episode of unusual severity. Maintenance therapy may include antidepressants for those bipolar patients who in their mixed phase require treatment of depressive symptomatology.

Schizoaffective and Schizophrenic Disorders. In patients with schizoaffective disorder, the combined use of lithium and a neuroleptic is often effective. This is particularly so in those patients who have a predominance of mood symptoms. Lithium is less effective in those schizoaffective disorders with a predominance of schizophrenic symptomatologies. Lithium does not appear to have exceptional efficacy in the treatment of uncomplicated schizophrenia and is rarely used for this purpose.

Cautions

The side effects of lithium are usually dose-dependent and are more likely to occur with dosages that exceed the usual therapeutic range. GI side effects in particular appear to be related to the degree of peak serum concentrations.

Nervous System Effects. Muscle weakness, tremor, lethargy, and, occasionally, fatigue may occur in close to half of all patients when they initially receive lithium. Mental confusion, dulled cognitive capabilities, and minor impairment of memory may also occur in up to one-third of patients. The tremor associated with lithium administration usually occurs at the time of drug initiation. It is a fine, rapid, intention tremor. A coarse tremor is usually associated with lithium toxicity. When severe it can be treated with β-adrenergic blocking agents. Fasciculations and clonic movements along with hyperactive reflexes may occur in some patients. Muscle weakness may occur.

GI Effects. Anorexia, nausea, vomiting, diarrhea, and abdominal pain may occur in up to one-third of patients. These usually occur at the time of drug initiation or drug increase and are associated with high peak serum concentrations of lithium. They can be reduced by administering the drug in divided doses and administering the drug with food. Occasionally it is necessary to switch a patient to a slow-release preparation.

Renal Effects. Polydipsia and polyuria occur in anywhere from one-third to one-half of patients taking lithium carbonate. These features usually develop at the time of drug initiation. They may persist in one-fourth of patients on long-term treatment. The polydipsia usually develops because of the polyuria. Dry mouth may also occur because of the polyuria.

Endocrine Effects. Hypothyroidism is the most common endocrinologic complication and occurs in approximately 4% of patients receiving long-term administration of lithium. Some cases of hypothyroidism may be severe enough to warrant exogenous thyroid supplementation. Goiters may also occur. These arise from thyroid gland stimulation produced by lithium-induced increase in thyrotropin release. In the majority of patients, however, there is only laboratory evidence of hypothyroidism with low T_4 and T_3 levels along with elevated thyroid-stimulating hormone (TSH) levels. Hyperparathyroidism may also occur, as may transient hyperglycemia.

Cardiovascular Effects. T wave inversion may occur. More commonly, T wave depression occurs. The latter finding is seen in approximately one-third of patients. It is benign and reversible. Sinus bradycardia, sinoatrial (SA) block, and AV node dissociation, with AV block and junctional rhythms and premature ventricular contractions, may rarely occur. Mild to moderate edema may occur.

Dermatologic Effects. The most common dermatologic side effects are acneiform eruptions and folliculitis. These usually respond to drug discontinuation. A pruritic maculopapular rash may also occur which likewise responds to dose reduction or discontinuation. Lithium may induce or exacerbate psoriasis. It may also produce drying of the skin.

Hematologic Effects. Lithium-induced leukocytosis is reversible and is usually in the range of 10,000 to 15,000/mm^3.

Other Adverse Effects. Long-term lithium use is associated with weight gain.

Precautions and Contraindications

For all patients taking lithium there should be regular monitoring of serum concentrations, clinical status, and thyroid hormone concentrations. Dosing needs to be adjusted in many cases as the patient's mania begins to abate. The patient's tolerance and need for higher doses of lithium will diminish along with the symptoms of mania. Dehydration poses a risk for patients of lithium toxicity. For this reason they should report nausea, vomiting, fever, diaphoresis, and polyuria to their physician. Patients should, in warm weather, maintain adequate hydration and sodium intake. Both salt intake and fluid intake should be increased in periods of fever. In many cases during periods of nausea, vomiting, diarrhea, fever, or polyuria, the lithium may need to be discontinued.

Lithium should be used with caution in patients who are sodium-restricted. Signs of lithium intoxication such as a muscle-twitching tremor, mild ataxia, muscle weakness, vomiting, diarrhea, and drowsiness should alert the patient and family to contact the physician and discontinue lithium therapy immediately.

Lithium should be used cautiously in patients with pre-existing thyroid disease.

Pregnancy, Fertility, and Lactation. A careful assessment of the risks and benefits must be made prior to the administration of lithium in pregnant females. Lithium may produce toxicity to the fetus, in particular. During the first trimester the drug may be associated with Ebstein's anomaly. This is a malformation of the tricuspid valve with secondary dilation of the right ventricular outflow tract. The period of greatest risk for this is during the first trimester. In neonates lithium exposure may produce hypotonia and apnea. Lithium is not known to have an impact on human fertility. Lithium is distributed into human breast milk. In general, lactating females on lithium should provide formula to their infants. During pregnancy careful monitoring of serum levels is required because of the changes in renal clearance and volume of distribution which occur during pregnancy and in the immediate postpartum period.

In general, clinicians reduce the dose of lithium in the week preceding the expected birth or when labor begins.

Chronic Toxicity

Pathogenesis. Chronic lithium toxicity is associated with high serum levels for prolonged periods of time. The most common cause of these high levels is water loss, often due to fever, vomiting, diarrhea, or diuretic use. Serum levels of 1.5 to 2.5 mEq/L represent moderate intoxication, 2.5 to 3.5 mEq/L indicates severe intoxication, and levels above 3.5 mEq/L are usually fatal.

Manifestations. Lithium intoxication initially presents with drowsiness, giddiness, apathy, confusion, coarse tremor, and dysarthria. GI symptoms such as vomiting, nausea, and diarrhea may be present. There may be muscle fasciculations, progressing to coarse and irregular tremors or choreoathetoid movements. Impaired consciousness, coma, seizures, and cardiovascular collapse may occur prior to death.

Treatment. Treatment is generally supportive. Lithium should be discontinued, and fluid and electrolyte abnormalities should be corrected. A diuretic may be administered in more severe cases along with intravenous (IV) infusion of 0.9% sodium chloride. Hemodialysis is begun when serum concentrations exceed 3 mEq/L, or at lower levels when the patient's condition is deteriorating; when fluid and electrolyte abnormalities do not respond to treatment; or when the serum lithium level is not falling in response to treatment.

The goal of hemodialysis should be to lower the serum level to less than 1 mEq/L after hemodialysis is completed. As mentioned, peritoneal dialysis is less effective than hemodialysis.

Acute Toxicity

See Chronic Toxicity above.

Pathogenesis. Acute lithium intoxication occurs after ingestion of a single dose of lithium that produces lithium concentrations greater than 3.5 mEq/L.

Treatment. The stomach should be emptied by gastric lavage or emesis. Subsequently, the treatment described above for chronic intoxication should be implemented.

Drug Interactions With Lithium

The interactions involving lithium and other drugs primarily occur at two levels: renal excretion, and direct receptor interaction (Table 3–2). Lithium carbonate, a salt of the alkali metal lithium, is neither protein-bound nor metabolized by the liver; it is filtered, reabsorbed, and excreted by the kidneys. For this reason, the most common cause of significant drug-drug interactions in patients receiving lithium are medications that affect the rate of renal clearance of lithium, thereby changing the plasma concentration (level) of lithium. The interaction effect on central and peripheral receptor sites of combining lithium with other medications is also clinically significant. Some medications work synergistically with lithium to produce an enhanced therapeutic effect in patients with bipolar affective disorder. The risk of neurotoxicity is also increased by an additive effect. The pharmacokinetics of lithium are closely related to the physiology of sodium, chloride, potassium, and fluid balance. Sodium depletion resulting from a salt-poor diet or diuretic regimen will decrease lithium clearance, thereby increasing the plasma Li^+ level and the potential risk of lithium toxicity. Also, hypokalemia, which may occur during the course of diuretic therapy, enhances the potential toxicity of lithium. The geriatric population and patients with renal disease are at increased risk for adverse effects from the combination of lithium with other medications.

Diuretics, Nonsteroidal Anti-inflammatory Agents, and Digoxin. Some drugs produce a definite reduction in renal excretion of lithium, thus increasing plasma Li^+ levels. These include thiazide diuretics, amiloride, furosemide, spironolactone, triamterene, and the nonsteroidal anti-inflammatory drugs (e.g., indomethacin and phenylbutazone, but not aspirin). Other drugs that may have the same effect are ibuprofen, naproxen, piroxicam, sulindac, and zomepirac. Some drugs reduce lithium levels by increasing the renal lithium excretion. These include acetazolamide, aminophylline, mannitol, sodium bicarbonate, sodium chloride, theophylline, and urea.

Patients receiving vigorous diuretic regimens for acute congestive heart failure or other serious conditions may require temporary discontinuance of lithium, particularly when hypokalemia occurs during the course of diuretic therapy. Lithium dosage reduction or temporary discontinuance is strongly recommended if lithium is being administered concurrently. Hypokalemia not only potentiates lithium toxicity but also significantly increases the risk of digitalis intoxication. Hypokalemia and digitalis toxicity may enhance the arrhythmogenic potential of lithium even when the latter is maintained at therapeutic serum levels. One report suggests that the therapeutic response to lithium is impaired during digoxin therapy.

Antipsychotics (Neuroleptics). Extensive use of the lithium-neuroleptic combination has generally proved quite safe and beneficial for manic patients; however, several reports have drawn attention to possible neurotoxic reactions following the combined use of lithium and neuroleptics (haloperidol, thioridazine, and chlorpromazine). Many of the signs and symptoms of the neurotoxic syndromes described are well-known toxic or side effects of either lithium or neuroleptics. However, it remains unclear whether such toxicity is unique secondary to lithium-neuroleptics per se. The few case reports of neurotoxicity associated with combined lithium and neuroleptics use do not permit generalization.

A review of 425 patients treated simultaneously with lithium and haloperidol failed to provide confirmation of toxic syndromes. It would be injudicious to discourage its combination, but it should undoubtedly be recognized that the combined use of lithium and a neuroleptic drug may have an idiosyncratic neurotoxic interaction. Patients treated under such conditions should be observed closely, and excessive dosages of either drug should be avoided.

Neuromuscular Blocking Agents, Electroconvulsive Therapy (ECT). Prolongation of muscle paralysis has been reported in lithium-treated patients who have received pancuronium and succinylcholine as muscle relaxants during the course of anesthesia. The mechanism appears to be a synergistic effect at the neuromuscular junction. These drug combinations may possibly have been used often during ECT with anesthesia and neuromuscular blockade. If so, it provides a relative contraindication to treatment with lithium during a course of ECT. Several reports show that ECT in patients taking lithium can occasionally lead to confusion, aggravated memory impairment, and seizure activity. It is advisable to discontinue lithium 3 to 5 days before the start of ECT until 1 to 2 days after the last treatment.

Iodide Salts or Thyroid Drugs. An antithyroid effect of lithium has now been generally recognized. Based on case reports, lithium and iodine may have an additive or synergistic effect in causing hypothyroidism. If patients receiving lithium become hypothyroid, the role of iodine from diet, proprietary medicines, and other sources should be investigated.

Anticonvulsants. CBZ may enhance the therapeutic effect of lithium in the treatment of mania. (For the interaction between CBZ and lithium, see under Carbamazepine above.) Although there have been case reports that suggest phenytoin combined with lithium may increase the risk of lithium-type toxicity, the toxicity may occur despite therapeutic lithium and phenytoin levels. In many, if not most cases, the drugs can be safely coadministered under careful supervision.

Miscellaneous Drugs. There have been four case reports suggesting increasing neurotoxicity in patients on lithium and methyldopa. Most of them were associated with therapeutic lithium levels. Patients taking both methyldopa and lithium should be closely monitored on the initiation and discontinuation of methyldopa. Based on case reports, the calcium channel blockers such as diltiazem and verapamil when given with lithium may provoke neurotoxic symptoms of lithium without an associated increased serum lithium concentration.

Table 3–2.
Drug Interactions With Lithium Carbonate

Combination	Interaction	Mechanism/ Comment	Clinical Significance
Antibiotics, e.g., tetracycline (oral), spectinomycin	↑ Plasma lithium level (in a few cases)	? ↓ Lithium clearance Case reports	?
Antidepressants			
Monoamine oxidase inhibitors (MAOIs)	↑ Antidepressant effect	Useful in treating severe or refractory depression	Yes
	Tardive dyskinesia?	Case reports, on long-term lithium-tranylcypromine treatment	?
Cyclic antidepressants	↑ Antidepressant effect ↓ Lower seizure threshold	Useful in treating refractory depression (? ↑ CNS serotonergic activity)	Yes
	Additive antithyroid effect	Case reports	Yes
Fluoxetine (Prozac)	↑ Plasma lithium levels?	Case report	?
Antihypertensives (nonthiazides)			
Clonidine	↓ Antihypertensive effects post chronic lithium treatment	? ↓ α_2 -Adrenergic receptor sensitivity (case report)	?
Angiotensin converting enzyme inhibitors, e.g., enalapril (Vasotec), captopril	↑ Lithium toxicity and ECG changes	↓ Lithium clearance? (sodium depletion) Case reports	?

Methyldopa	↑ Neurotoxicity in a few cases (in a few cases)	Intoxication may occur even though lithium levels are within therapeutic range Avoid this combination Replacement by β-blocker is advisable	Yes
Antipsychotics (neuroleptics), e.g., haloperidol, phenothiazines	Worsen lithium neurotoxicity/ extrapyramidal symptoms (especially haloperidol, thioridazine)	Mechanism ? Case reports	?
	↓↓ Chlorpromazine (CPZ) plasma concentration (up to 50%–60%)	↑ CPZ excretion Acute lithium withdrawal may cause CPZ intoxication	Yes
	? Hyperglycemia	Case reports ? Mechanism Management of neurotoxic extra-pyramidal syndromes: discontinue neuroleptics and reduce lithium dosage	?
Benzodiazepines	? Hypothermia	Mechanism? Single case report (diazepam)	?
Carbamazepine	Enhance lithium effect	Synergistic effect	Yes
	Possible ↑ risk of neurotoxicity?	? Mechanism ? Idiosyncratic reaction	Yes

(Continued.)

Table 3–2 (cont.).

Combination	Interaction	Mechanism/ Comment	Clinical Significance
		Patients with underlying systemic medical illness or concurrently use of other drugs may be predisposed to risk, when treated with this combination	
Cisplatin	↓ Plasma lithium levels	? Mechanism	Yes
Diclofenac (Voltarol, Voltaren) furosemide	↓ Renal clearance of lithium (↑ plasma lithium levels)	? Mechanism Clinical trials suggest	Yes
Digoxin	↑ Risk of digoxin toxicity ↓ Lithium therapeutic effect	↓ Intracellular potassium Suggested by case report	? ?
Diuretics			
Carbonic anhydrase inhibitors: acetazolamide (Diamox), etc.	↓ Plasma lithium levels	↑ Lithium excretion (impairs proximal tubular reabsorption of lithium)	Yes
Loop diuretics: bumetanide (Bumex), furosemide (Lasix), ethacrynic acid (Edecrin)	↑ Plasma lithium levels	? Mechanism (↑ sodium depletion?) Evidence not well established Closely monitor signs and symptoms of lithium toxicity	?

Osmotic diuretics (e.g., mannitol)	↓ Plasma lithium levels	↑ Lithium excretion Has been used in the treatment of lithium intoxication	Yes
Potassium-sparing diuretics (e.g., spironolactone, triameterene, amiloride)	↑ Plasma lithium levels	↑ Tubular reabsorption	Yes
Thiazide diuretics (e.g., bendroflumethiazide)	↑ Plasma lithium levels	↑ Tubular reabsorption (↓ renal lithium clearance)	Yes
Xanthine diuretics (aminophylline, caffeine, theophylline)	↓ Plasma lithium levels	↑ Lithium excretion (related to theophylline serum levels?) Clinical trial	Yes
Ethanol	↓ Alcohol withdrawal?	Clinical implication?	?
Hydroxyzine	Cardiac conduction disturbance	↑ Effect of lithium on cardiac repolarization? Case report	?
Iodine salts, e.g., potassium iodide (SSK)	↑ Hypothyroidism	Lithium blocks both uptake of iodine into thyroid gland and release of thyroid hormone; potassium iodide inhibits thyroid hormone synthesis	Yes
q		↑ Have clinical value in treating thyrotoxicosis	Yes

(Continued.)

Table 3–2 (cont.).

Combination	Interaction Effects	Mechanism/ Comment	Clinical Significance
Ketamine	↑ Length of ketamine anesthesia	Mechanism: unknown	?
Levodopa	↑ Mental and motor side effects of levodopa	Mechanism? Controversial reports	?
Marijuana	↑ Plasma lithium levels	Mechanism? Case report	?
Mazindol	↑ Plasma lithium levels (lithium toxicity)	Single case report may be associated with salt-poor diet	?
Nonsteroidal antiinflammatory drugs (NSAIDs), e.g., diclofenac (Voltaren), ibuprofen (Motrin), indomethacin (Indocin), naproxen (Anaprox, Naprosyn), piroxicam (Feldene), sulindac	↑ Plasma lithium levels (↑ therapeutic and toxic effects of lithium)	Mechanism? (↓ renal clearance of lithium via prostaglandin-dependent mechanism?) Aspirin does not alter lithium clearance Closely monitor lithium levels and tailor dosage is if an NSAID is added	Yes
Neuromuscular blocking agents depolarizing group: succinylcholine (Anectine)	↑ Neuromuscular blocking effects	Mechanism? (inhibition of serum cholinesterase activity?)	Yes
Nondepolarizing group: e.g., tubocurarine, gallamine, triethiodide (Flaxedil), pancuronium (Pavulon)	↑ Neuromuscular blocking effects (↑ respiratory depression)	One report inconsistent with this result	

		Mechanism ? Possibly affects (↓) acetylcholine activity at nerve terminals Tailor dosage of neuromuscular blocking agents and provide life support if needed	Yes
Phenytoin	Neurotoxicity	Mechanism? May occur despite therapeutic lithium and phenytoin levels Case reports	
Sodium chloride	↓ Plasma lithium levels	↑ Lithium excretion	Yes
Sympathomimetic, parenteral, e.g., norepinephrine (Levophed), phenylephrine (Neo-Synephrine)	↓ Pressor sensitivity	Mechanism?	?
Urea	↓ Plasma lithium levels	↑ Lithium excretion Single study of 6 subjects with higher urea dosage	?
Urinary alkalinizers (e.g., sodium bicarbonate)	↓ Plasma lithium levels	↓ Lithium clearance Sodium bicarbonate is a component of some over-the-counter antacids	Yes
Verapamil, diltiazem	↑ Lithium toxicity (without elevated plasma lithium levels)	Synergistic effects 2 case reports have shown conflicting data: (↓ plasma lithium levels, mechanism?)	Yes

Dosage and Administration

Dosage. The individual dosage should be titrated to the appropriate serum levels. Individual needs vary widely. Serum levels should be determined approximately 12 hours after the last oral dose. Levels of 1.0 to 1.4 mEq/L are usually used for acute manic treatment. Levels ranging from 0.6 to 1.0 mEq/L are usually used for long-term treatment. The initial dosage may range anywhere from 300 to 600 mg three times a day. Side effects are more common with higher serum levels and compliance more problematic. Dosage should be titrated to an individual's need, clinical response, and tolerance.

Maintenance Dosage. Most clinicians maintain patients in the range of 0.6 to 1.0 mEq/L and attempt to minimize side effects.

Administration. There does not appear to be a significant difference in the bioavailability of the various lithium preparations. Lithium citrate is helpful in patients unable to swallow oral capsules or tablets. Lithium citrate 8 mEq is approximately equivalent to 300 mg of lithium carbonate. The hallmark of good lithium therapy is careful frequent monitoring of serum lithium concentrations and monitoring of the patient's clinical status for both symptomatic improvement and the development of side effects. During initial lithium administration, levels are monitored frequently, usually every 5 days. Thereafter, levels may be monitored every 1 to 2 months for the first 6 months and subsequently every 3 to 6 months for long-term use. Significant changes in the clinical condition warrant repeat checking of the serum levels.

Preparations

Lithium carbonate
- Oral capsules (*Eskalith, Lithonate*)
  - 150 mg (4.06 mEq), 300 mg (8.12 mEq), 600 mg (16.24 mEq)
- Tablets (*Eskalith Lithane*)
  - 300 mg (8.12 mEq)
- Tablets, extended-release (*Eskalith*)
  - 450 mg (12.18 mEq)
- Tablets, extended-release, film-coated (*Lithobid*)
  - 300 mg (8.12 mEq)
- Tablets, film coated (*Lithotabs*)
  - 300 mg (8.12 mEq)

Lithium citrate
Oral solution (*Cibalith-S Syrup*)
8 mEq/5 mL

VALPROATE SODIUM, VALPROIC ACID, DIVALPROEX SODIUM

Pharmacology

The mechanism of action of valproic acid (VPA) is unknown but is believed to be in part due to increased concentrations of γ-aminobutyric acid (GABA). The concentrations of the inhibitory neurotransmitter are raised by VPA as a result of inhibition of GABA metabolism.

Pharmacokinetics

Absorption. VPA is rapidly and almost completely absorbed from the GI tract. When taken with meals its absorption is somewhat delayed. Valproate sodium is rapidly converted to VPA in the stomach. Divalproex sodium dissociates into valproate which is then absorbed. Divalproex sodium has the same bioavailability as valproate.

Distribution. VPA is found in breast milk and crosses the placenta. It is also found in other exchangeable extracellular water such as CSF and saliva. It is rapidly distributed after absorption and is bound to plasma proteins.

Elimination. VPA has an average half-life of 10 hours. There is, however, a wide variability among patients. VPA is metabolized in the liver via oxidation, with metabolites being excreted in the urine.

Uses

VPA, valproate sodium, and divalproex sodium have been found to be effective in the management of acute mania.

Cautions

GI Effects. Frequently nausea, vomiting, and indigestion complicate the administration of VPA. Usually these effects are short term and are minimized by administering the drug with meals and using the lowest possible doses to initiate therapy. Divalproex sodium appears to have the lowest incidence of adverse GI effects.

Less commonly, changes in appetite including increased appetite with weight gain, cramps, diarrhea, or constipation and hypersalivation or anorexia with weight loss may occur with the administration of VPA.

Nervous Systems Effects. Patients should be cautioned about engaging in activities which require mental alertness such as operating machinery or driving vehicles since VPA may produce sedation and drowsiness. Other less common effects include ataxia, nystagmus, tremor, dizziness, and dysarthria.

Hepatic Effects. Dose-related elevations in lactate dehydrogenase and aminotransferases, usually of a minor nature, may occur. Less commonly, liver function tests including serum bilirubin may show increased values, indicating serious hepatotoxicity. Severe hepatic complications are most common in children under 2 years of age taking other anticonvulsants. The frequency of fatal hepatotoxicity decreases with increasing age. In most cases it is preceded by a general malaise, weakness, anorexia, vomiting, and lethargy.

Metabolic Effects. Abnormal elevations in serum ammonia concentrations may occur with or without lethargy and may occur in the presence of normal hepatic function tests.

Hematologic Effects. There have been reports of bone marrow depression and its concomitant clinical manifestations. VPA may also prolong the bleeding time.

Pregnancy, Fertility, and Lactation. The safety of VPA administration during pregnancy has not been established. A causal relationship between the administration of VPA to pregnant women and an increased incidence of birth defects has not been established. However, there is a suspicion that VPA may produce neural tube defects and for this reason it should be used with caution in women of childbearing age and should only be administered to pregnant women when the benefits clearly outweigh the risks. Caution should be exercised in lactating women since VPA is distributed into breast milk. Lactating women should be advised to discontinue nursing and use formula.

Precautions and Contraindications

VPA may cause a potentially fatal hepatotoxicity. For this reason baseline hepatic function tests should be obtained prior to drug initiation. Furthermore, they should be repeated at regular intervals during drug therapy, in particular, during the first 6 months of drug administration. In fact, VPA should be discontinued promptly when there is evidence of hepatic dysfunction. In some cases the liver dysfunction will progress despite discontinuation of the drug. VPA should not be used in patients with hepatic disease, a history of hepatic disease, or substantial hepatic dysfunction. If hyperammonemia occurs the drug should be discontinued. If clinical evidence of bone marrow depression, including hemorrhage, bruising, or a disorder of coagulation, develops, VPA should be discontinued.

Acute Toxicity

Manifestations and Treatment. Overdosage may produce sedation or coma. Treatment is supportive. It is important to maintain adequate urinary output to enhance drug excretion. In general, gastric lavage is of little use because of the rapid drug absorption.

Drug Interactions with Valproic Acid

Several reports suggest that the potential for VPA toxicity may be increased during *aspirin-VPA* coadministration. The combination of VPA and CBZ resulted in higher plasma levels of the CBZ active metabolite CBZ 10,11-epoxide, while CBZ levels were not significantly affected, or were reduced at various levels. VPA also may cause protein binding displacement of CBZ. Theoretically there is the possibility that CBZ intoxication may develop when using these medications in combination. Additional impairment in consciousness may occur when other central nervous system (CNS) depressants are coadministered with VPA. These include alcohol and other anticonvulsants. VPA may potentiate the effects of MAOIs and other antidepressants. For this reason dosages of these drugs may need to be reduced when VPA is administered to these patients. VPA appears to impair the metabolism of phenobarbital and increase plasma phenobarbital levels. Clinical studies suggest that phenytoin may in some but not all cases increase the metabolism of VPA when the two drugs are coadministered. In addition, phenytoin levels may decrease transiently when VPA is added, although the evidence is contradictory. Chlorpromazine may competitively inhibit the metabolism of VPA and decrease the clearance of VPA, which may lead to VPA toxicity. There is an increase in the unbound fraction of thiopentone in rabbits also receiving VPA. Unbound thiopentone would be more accessible to the CNS leading to prolonged hypnotic anesthetic effects. The drug interactions with VPA are summarized in Table 3–3.

Dosage and Administration

Dosage. Dosage should be titrated slowly and in response to the patient's tolerance and needs. A general dose should be administered in two or more divided doses. The usual starting dose is 15 mg/kg/day and is increased by 5 to 10 mg/kg/day at weekly intervals.

Administration. VPA, divalproex sodium, and valproate sodium are administered orally. Divalproex sodium may be less likely to produce GI side effects.

Preparations

Valproate sodium (*Depa Syrup, Depakene Syrup, Myproic Acid Syrup*)
  Oral solution
    250 mg/5 mL
Valproic acid (*Depakene*)
  Oral capsules
    250 mg
Divalproex sodium (*Depakote*)
  Oral tablets, enteric-coated
    125 mg, 250 mg, 500 mg

VERAPAMIL HYDROCHLORIDE

Pharmacology

Verapamil is a calcium channel blocking agent. As such, its principle physiologic action is the inhibition of the flux of extracellular calcium ions across the membrane of myocardial cells and vascular smooth muscle cells without changing serum calcium concentrations. The exact mechanism that verapamil uses to inhibit calcium ion influx across slow calcium channels is unknown, but may involve the inhibition of ion-controlled gating mechanisms of the channel, or by deforming the slow channel, or by interfering with the release of calcium from the sarcoplasmic reticulum, or by any of these in combination.

Verapamil inhibits coronary artery spasm in patients with vasospastic angina. It decreases peripheral vascular resistance and has inhibitory effects on the cardiac conduction system.

Verapamil reduces myocardial contractility.

Pharmacokinetics

Absorption. Approximately 90% of an orally administered dose is rapidly absorbed from the GI tract following oral administration of conventional tablets. However, there is extensive first-pass metabolism resulting in only 20% to 35% of an oral dose reaching the systemic circulation.

Distribution. Approximately 90% of verapamil is bound to plasma proteins. Verapamil distributes into the CNS with approximately 6% of the administered dose reaching the CSF and 4% of its active primary metabolite being detectable in the CSF.

Elimination. Verapamil has a half-life of approximately 2 to 8 hours. After approximately 1 to 2 days of administration, however, the half-life may increase to 4.5 to 12 hours. This is thought to be due to saturation of the hepatic enzymes.

Verapamil is metabolized in the liver. Norverapamil is an active metabolite.

Cautions

Verapamil is usually well tolerated in conventional dosages. However, in approximately 6% of all patients adverse effects may require a reduction in the dosage and in approximately 5% of patients adverse effects may require discontinuation of the drug. The incidence and severity of adverse effects are more common with IV administration.

Cardiovascular Effects. Serious adverse effects occur in approximately 2% of patients and may include bradycardia, first, second, or third degree AV block, AV dissociation, and bundle-branch block.

GI Effects. Constipation occurs in approximately 9% of patients, and nausea and GI discomfort in approximately 3%.

Nervous System Effects. Four percent of patients may develop dizziness, and headache and fatigue are seen in approximately 2%.

Hepatic Effects. Transient increases in aspartate aminotransferase (AST, SGOT) and alanine aminotransferase (ALT, SGPT), with or without concomitant increases in alkaline phosphatase and bilirubin, may occur. Periodic monitoring of liver function tests are recommended as are baseline liver function studies.

Precautions and Contraindications. IV verapamil should be used only in a hospital setting where an ECG and hemodynamic

Table 3–3.
Drug Interactions With Valproic Acid (VPA) or Sodium Valproate

Combination	Interaction	Mechanism/ Comment	Clinical Significance
Aspirin	↑ Free fraction of VPA and potential toxicity of VPA (tremor, drowsiness, ataxia, nystagmus, personality changes)	Salicylates displace VPA from its plasma protein binding site Inhibits β-oxidation of VPA	Yes
Barbiturates (phenobarbital, primidone)	↑ Barbiturate plasma level	↓ Hepatic degradation of barbiturates	Yes
Carbamazepine	↓ VPA levels with possible loss of seizure control Variable changes in CBZ concentrations with ↑ levels of CBZ active metabolite 10, 11-epoxide	Multiple mechanisms are probably involved (CBZ ↑ VPA clearance, and VPA inhibits metabolism of 10, 11-epoxide)	Yes
Cimetidine	↑ Half-life and ↓ clearance of VPA	Mechanism ? When adding or removing cimetidine from regimen of a patients receiving VPA, monitor serum levels of VPA and clinical signs and symptoms of side effects or epileptic breakthrough	?
Clonazepam (Clonopin)	Severe drowsiness and loss of seizure control	Mechanism ?	?

		Case report proposed; clinical investigations fail to demonstrate similar reactions	?
Diazepam	↑ Level of unbound plasma diiazepam and ↓ serum level of diazepam metabolite	VPA displaces diazepam from plasma protein binding sites and inhibits its metabolism	?
Hydantoins: phenytoin (Dilantin)	↓ Pharmacologic effects of VPA	Phenytoin increases hepatic metabolism of VPA	Yes
	Variable change in phenytoin serum concentration (decrease, increase, no changes)	VPA competes with phenytoin for serum protein binding	
		Observe patient for phenytoin toxicity or loss of seizure control	
Isoniazid	↑ Toxic effects of both drugs	? Mechanism	?
		Single case report	
Phenothiazine, chlorpromazine (Thorazine)	↓ Clearance of VPA	Possibly inhibitionn of VPA metabolism	?
Succinimides: ethosuximide (ESM, Zarontin)	Variable changes in ESM levels (increased, decreased, no change)	↑ ESM concentration is probably due to VPA inhibition of ESM metabolism	?
		Inhibition of ESM metabolism by VPA only presents a problem when other antiepileptic drugs are also being used, competing for the enzyme systems	

monitoring and resuscitative equipment are available during the initial stages of treatment.

Likewise, because of its tendency to lower peripheral vascular resistance and occasionally produce symptomatic hypotension, blood pressure should be monitored carefully.

Verapamil should be used with caution in patients with ventricular dysfunction or heart failure and in patients with hepatic or renal impairment.

Acute Toxicity

Manifestations. Overdosage of verapamil produces signs and symptoms that are extensions of common adverse reactions.

Treatment. Treatment is generally supportive, but, in some cases β-adrenergic agonists and IV calcium salts may be useful. Clinically important hypotension should be treated with an IV calcium salt or vasopressor agent (e.g., norepinephrine).

Drug Interactions With Verapamil

Cardiac Drugs. In hypertension and unstable angina, combined β-blocker and verapamil therapy is generally effective and acceptable, but the pharmacologic and adverse effects of certain β-blockers and verapamil may be increased. It may cause profound untoward cardiovascular effects in some patients (e.g., SA node disease, AV conduction defects, and heart failure). Verapamil has markedly increased the plasma levels of metoprolol but not atenolol, while minimally affecting propranolol levels. However, one study has shown that chronic verapamil administration may increase steady-state atenolol plasma levels. Digoxin and digitoxin plasma levels may be increased by verapamil. Toxicity may result, characterized by GI and neuropsychiatric symptoms and cardiac arrhythmias. Adequate digoxin and digitoxin dosage reduction are recommended to avoid unnecessary risk during the coadministration. A series of studies has demonstrated an increase in both hypotensive effects and prazosin serum concentrations when prazosin is coadministered with verapamil. Though verapamil and quinidine have been used together successfully, significant adverse reactions from the combination have been reported. Concomitant use of oral verapamil and quinidine resulted in marked hypotension, bradycardia, ventricular tachycardia, AV block, and pulmonary edema in a small number of patients with hypertrophic cardiomyopathy.

Table 3–4.
Drug Interactions With Verapamil

Combination	Interaction Effects	Mechanism/ Comment	Clinical Significance
Barbiturates: (phenobarbital, etc.)	↓ Pharmacologic effects of of verapamil	↑ Verapamil first-pass hepatic metabolism If an interaction is suspected, consider increasing the dose of verapamil	?
β-Blockers: atenolol (Tenormin), metoprolol (Lopressor), Pindolol (Visken), Propranolol (Inderal), timolol (Biocadren)	Pharmacologic and adverse effects of β-blockers and verapamil may be increased	Synergistic or addictive cardiovascular effects (?) (both have negative chronotropic and inotropic effects) If adverse cardia effects appear, lower the dose of either drug β_1-selective agents may be preferable	Yes
Calcium salt, vitamin D	↓ Clinical effects and toxicity of verapamil	Pharmacologic antagonism Calcium has been used to treat verapamil toxicity	Yes
Cimetidine	? ↑ Verapamil oral bioavailability and half-life	Inhibition of verapamil metabolism Conflicting data: some studies were unable to provide evidence of interaction	?
Carbamazepine (see Table 2–1)			

(Continued.)

Table 3–4 (cont.).

Combination	Interaction Effects	Mechanism/ Comment	Clinical Significance
Cyclosporine (SANDIMMUNE)	↑ Cyclosporine levels and potential nephrotoxicity	? Inhibition of cyclosporine metabolism Administration of verapamil before cyclosporine may be nephroprotective (?) Nifedipine may decrease cyclosporine nephrotoxicity (?)	?
Digitoxin, digoxin	↑ Digitoxin and digoxin serum levels; toxicity may result (e.g., GI and neuropsychiatric symptoms and cardiac arrhythmias) Additive depression of cardiac conduction may occur	? Mechanism Monitor for clincial signs of digitoxin/digoxin efficacy/toxicity and serum levels Tailor digitoxin/digoxin doses as needed	Yes
Glibenclamide (glyburide)	↑ Plasma levels of glibenclamide	Mechanism? No effect on plasma glucose or insulin	?
Lithium (see Table 3–2)			
Muscle relaxants Nondepolarizing group: pancuronium (Pavulon), tubocurarine, vecuronium	↑ Neuromuscular blocking effects	Verapamil blocks pre- and postjunctional calcium channels Avoid this combination If necessary, tailor muscle relaxant	Yes

(Norcuron)		dosage and monitor respiratory function closely; provide mechanical ventilatory support	
Prazosin (Minipress)	↑ Prazosin serum concentration ↑ Sensitivity to prazosin-induced postural hypotension	Mechanism? Rapid onset If combined therapy is necessary, advise patient to take precautions regarding postural hypotension	Yes
Quinidine (Cin-Quin)	Hypotension, bradycardia, ventricular tachycardia, AV block, pulmonary edema	Verapamil may interfere with clearance of quinidine and prolong half-life Avoid combined use in IHSS patients Management: a. Monitor patients closely b. Stop one, or both of the drugs if the interaction appears c. Symptomatic treatment	Yes
Rifampin	↓ Pharmacologic effects of oral verapamil	↑ First-pass hepatic metabolism Effects may persist for several days after discontinuing rifampin Minimal effects of rifampin on IV verapamil	Yes
Sulfinpyrazone (Anturane)	↓ Verapamil's therapeutic effects	↑ Metabolic clearance of Verapamil (?)	?
Theophylines: Theophyline (Bronkodyl)	↑ Action of theophylines	Mechanism ? Nifedipine may decrease or have no effect on theophyline serum levels	?

Calcium salts and vitamin D may decrease the pharmacologic effects of verapamil. Calcium salts have been used successfully to treat verapamil toxicity. However, in two cases of severe verapamil poisoning, calcium gluconate improved arrhythmias but did not reverse hypotension or bradycardia. The effectiveness of such therapy may depend on factors such as the dose of each drug and the chronicity of verapamil use.

Miscellaneous Drugs. Rifampin may decrease the pharmacologic effects of oral verapamil. The effects may persist for several days after discontinuing rifampin. However, pharmacokinetic studies have demonstrated minimal effects of rifampin on IV verapamil. The effects of nondepolarizing muscle relaxants may be enhanced owing to verapamil's ability to block pre- and postjunctional calcium channels. Avoid this combination, but if necessary, tailor the dose of muscle relaxant, and monitor respiratory function closely. The pharmacologic effects or potential toxicity of CBZ may be increased owing to the inhibition of hepatic metabolism by verapamil and possibly by diltiazem. Coadministration of lithium and verapamil, causing both a reduction in lithium levels with decreased antimanic control and lithium toxicity, have been reported, and lithium plasma levels may not be predictive of such toxicity.

The drug interactions with verapamil are summarized in Table 3–4.

Dosage and Administration

Dosage. Dosage should be titrated to individual needs.

Administration. In psychiatric use verapamil is administered only orally.

Preparations

Verapamil hydrochloride

- Oral tablets, extended-release, film-coated (*Calan SR, Isoptin SR*)
  - 240 mg
- Oral tablets, film-coated (*Calan, Isoptin*)
  - 40 mg, 80 mg, 120 mg

BENZO-DIAZEPINES 4

GENERAL STATEMENT

The benzodiazepines share several properties, including their efficacy as anxiolytics, hypnotics, sedatives, anticonvulsants, and skeletal muscle relaxants. These effects of the benzodiazepines are caused by potentiation of an inhibitory neurotransmitter, γ-aminobutyric acid (GABA). These effects on GABA occur throughout the central nervous system (CNS), including the hypothalamus, and the limbic and thalamic regions of the brain. The benzodiazepines reduce the amount of rapid eye movement (REM) sleep. There is also a reduction in stage 3 and stage 4 sleep. The antiseizure effects of benzodiazepines appear to be caused by augmentation of presynaptic inhibitions. The CNS depressant effects are capable of producing a wide range of CNS depression ranging from mild sedation through sleep to coma.

Pharmacokinetics

Absorption. Benzodiazepines are well absorbed from the gastrointestinal (GI) tract following oral administration. Lorazepam is also well absorbed following intramuscular (IM) administration. Most benzodiazepines undergo extensive metabolism—many have active metabolites. Metabolism and serum levels of the benzodiazepines vary greatly among individuals. Many of the metabolites are physiologically active.

Distribution. Benzodiazepines are widely distributed in the CNS and most body fluids and tissues. In addition, these drugs are distributed into human breast milk; they also cross the placenta, and are found in the fetus.

Elimination. The half-lives of benzodiazepines and their metabolites vary widely among individuals. In general, the elderly and patients with renal disease have prolonged elimination of benzodiazepines with the exception of triazolam, oxazepam, temazepam, and lorazepam (all of which do not have active metabolites).

Half-lives for benzodiazepines are:

Drug	Half-Life (hr)	Half-Life of Active Metabolites (hr)
Alprazolam	12–15	
Chlordiazepoxide	5–30	24–96
Clonazepam	18–50	
Clorazepate	Rapidly metabolized	50–100
Diazepam	20–50	50–100
Flurazepam	2	74–160
Halazepam	14	50–100
Lorazepam	10–20	
Oxazepam	5–15	
Prazepam		50–100
Quazepam	39 hours	74–160
Temazepam	10–20	
Triazolam	1.5–5.0	

Alprazolam, clonazepam, lorazepam, oxazepam, temazepam, and triazolam do not have active metabolites. In the liver, oxazepam, lorazepam, temazepam, and the hydroxylated metabolites of clorazepate, chlordiazepoxide, diazepam, halazepam, flurazepam, prazepam, and triazolam are conjugated. These inactive conjugates are excreted in the urine.

Uses

Benzodiazepines are used in the treatment of anxiety, alcohol withdrawal, insomnia, muscle spasticity, seizure disorders, and as light anesthesia in surgery. In addition, they are effective when used in the treatment of mania in conjunction with lithium. All benzodiazepines appear to be approximately equally effective if an adequate dosage is given for these purposes. The major differences used to guide drug selection are the pharmacokinetic properties.

There is no established proof of the efficacy of benzodiazepines in the treatment of anxiety when they are administered for longer than 4 continuous months. In such instances, there should be a periodic reassessment of the need and efficacy of benzodiazepines.

Most clinicians consider benzodiazepines the drug of choice for inducing sleep; the efficacy of benzodiazepines for inducing sleep is well established for the first 2 to 4 weeks. Continued efficacy beyond that period of time has not been clearly established. As with the treatment of anxiety, with prolonged use of benzodiazepines for sleep induction, there should be periodic reassessment of their continued efficacy and need. In particular, triazolam, temazepam, quazepam, and flurazepam have been shown to be effective when administered for 1 month. A major concern with the use of benzodiazepines (or other sedatives) as hypnotics is that withdrawal insomnia will develop within 1 to 2 weeks of nightly use followed by termination of the drug. Drug tolerance may also develop during this time. Therefore, it may be best to encourage patients to limit drug use to two to three times per week to avoid the development of these problems.

Most clinicians consider benzodiazpines to be the medications of choice in the treatment of transient anxiety. When treating elderly patients, or those with hepatic disease, lorazepam or oxazepam may be preferable to other benzodiazepines because of their relatively short elimination half-life and the absence of active metabolites.

Cautions

CNS Effects. Adverse effects are more common during the initiation of therapy and tend to diminish with continued treatment. Debilitated patients, children, the elderly, and patients with hepatic or renal disease are more likely to experience CNS side effects. Their vulnerability to these effects can be minimized when lower initial drug dosages are provided. Common adverse effects include ataxia, drowsiness, confusion, weakness, fatigue, dizziness, and syncope. There may be headache, dysarthria, vivid dreams, and in the elderly, a reversible dementia. Encephalopathy may occur in patients with renal failure. Abrupt discontinuation may produce anxiety, disturbed sleep, and in some cases, seizures. Some individuals may develop a response consisting of general CNS stimulation; this is characterized by restlessness, anxiety, tremulousness, sleep disturbance, talkativeness, along with general hyperactivity and excitement. There may also be hyperreflexia and muscle spasticity.

Other Adverse Effects. Some patients receiving benzodiazepines may complain of changes in appetite, constipation, weight, libido, and menstrual irregularities, along with galactorrhea, gynecomastia, and failure to ovulate, have also been reported. Other complaints have included joint and body pain and paresthesias. There have been genitourinary complaints such as difficulty initiating urination and urinary incontinence. Some patients may develop photosensitivity and a rash. When benzodiazepines are administered parenterally, patients may develop apnea, hypotension, bradycardia, or cardiac arrest. These effects are more likely to occur in debilitated patients or the elderly. There have been reports of benzodiazepines producing elevations in serum lactate dehydrogenase (LDH), alanine (ALT, SGPT) and aspartate (AST, SGOT) aminotransferases, and, alkaline phosphatase, along with direct and total serum bilirubin.

Precautions and Contraindications. Because benzodiazepines may impair mental alertness and physical coordination, patients should be cautioned against engaging in hazardous activity which requires mental alertness or coordination, such as driving a motor vehicle or operating machinery. Certain individuals may be likely to abuse benzodiazepines. In particular, patients with a prior history of substance abuse or with significant personality disorders may be more vulnerable to escalate the dose on their own or to use the drug in suicide attempts. These populations should be assessed carefully prior to the administration of benzodiazepines.

Pregnancy, Fertility, and Lactation. The safety of benzodiazepines during the first trimester of pregnancy has not been fully established. Thus, most clinicians feel that the use of benzodiazepines as anxiolytics or hypnotics is contraindicated during pregnancy. Furthermore, the infants of mothers who receive chronic benzodiazepines during pregnancy may develop withdrawal symptoms after delivery. Women of childbearing potential should be cautioned about the hazards associated with becoming pregnant while on benzodiazepine treatment. Mothers of newborns who are nursing should be cautioned to avoid benzodiazepine use while nursing since benzodiazepines are distributed into human breast milk and cause toxicity in the infant.

Chronic Toxicity

Chronic use of benzodiazepines may lead to the development of psychological and physiologic dependence, and tolerance may develop. In patients who have received benzodiazepines on a chronic basis, abrupt withdrawal may produce a withdrawal syndrome which includes anxiety, loss of appetite, insomnia, sweating, diarrhea, irritability, vomiting, and a general dysphoria. There may be tremor, ataxic gait, muscle and abdominal cramps, and ultimately seizures. In mild cases there may simply be insomnia, anxiety, and general dysphoria.

Acute Toxicity

Overdosage may result in varying degrees of CNS depression including somnolence, confusion, coma, and ultimately hypotension, and respiratory depression may lead to death. However, in almost all cases death occurs when there is concurrent ingestion of alcohol or other CNS depressants. In general, during benzodiazepine overdosage, treatment is symptomatic and supportive. If the ingestion has been recent, the stomach should be emptied of any remaining drug by gastric lavage. There should be careful monitoring of pulse, blood pressure, and respiration along with maintenance of an adequate airway.

Drug Interactions

When the benzodiazepines are administered concomitantly with other CNS depressants there may be an additive CNS depressant effect. When alprazolam, chlordiazepoxide, diazepam, or triazolam are administered with cimetidine (or disulfiram, ethanol, or isoniazid) there may be increased plasma concentrations of the benzodiazepines because the latter drugs (cimetidine, etc.) reduce plasma clearance of benzodiazepines that undergo oxidative metabolism.

Table 4–1.
Drug Interactions With Benzodiazepines (BZDs)

Combination	Interaction Effects	Mechanism/ Comment	Clinical Significance
Antacids (aluminum hydroxide–containing) (e.g., Maalox, Gelusi) with diazepam, clorazepate, chlordiazepoxide	Decrease peak concentration and clinical effects of diazepam, etc.	Antacids reduce/delay rate of GI absorption of diazepam, etc. (but not amounts) No special precaution appears necessary	?
Antidepressants Tricyclic (TCA)-chlordiazepoxide Mongamine oxidase inhibitors (MAOIs), e.g., phenelzine (Nardil) with chlordiazepoxide, isocarboxazid (Marplan), chlordiazepoxide	May ↑ sedation or atropine-like effects Mass edema	Mechanism? (case report) It may occur with other BZD-TCA combinations No special precautions appear necessary	?
Cimetidine (Tagamet)-BZD (coxidation) (e.g., alprazolam, chlordiazepoxide, clorazepate, diazepam, flurazepam, midazolam [Versed], triazolam)	↑ Serum levels of some BZDs; certain actions, especially sedation, may be enhanced	Mechanism: Inhibition of hepatic oxidative metabolism (mainly) Reduction of presystemic metabolism as a result of reduced hepatic blood flow Monitor for increased/prolonged sedation during coadminstration	Yes

		Similar interaction has been reported between cimetidine and lorazepam (glucuronidation BZD) due to cimetidine reducing liver blood flow	
Contraceptives, oral BZD (oxidation)	May prolong BZD half-life ($t^1/_2$) and ↑ serum levels	Decrease in BZD oxidation rate; mechanism?	?
BZD (glucuronidation) (lorazepam, oxazepam, temazepam)	May ↑ BZD clearance rate	Reduction in BZD dosage may be required in some patients Increase rate of BZD glucuronidation; mechanism?	?
Dextropropoxyphene-alprazolam	May potentiate CNS depressant effects	↓ Clearance rate of alprazolam and synergistic effect By the same volunteer study, diazapram is less affected and there is no effect on lorazepam	Yes
Diflunisal (Dolobid)-oxazepam	May decrease bioavailibility of oxazepam	Diflunisal may displace oxazepam from protein binding sites (single-dose study)	?
Digoxin–diazepam, alprazolam	May increase digoxin serum concentrations and toxicity	Mechanism ? Routinely monitor digoxin levels during coadministration Conflicting data on digoxin-alprazolam interaction	?

(Continued.)

Table 4–1 (cont.).

Combination	Interaction Effects	Mechanism/ Comment	Clinical Significance
Diphenhydramine-temazepam	Stillbirth (caused by convulsion?)	Case report Avoid this combination during pregnancy	?
Disulfiram-BZD (oxidation)	May increase CNS depressant actions	Disulfiram may inhibit hepatic metabolism of BZDs that undergo oxidation	
Doxapram (Dopram)-Diazepam, etc.	Reverse sedation	Antagonistic effect Clinically useful interaction	Yes
Ethanol-BZD (chlordiazepoxide, diazepam, lorazepam, triazolam, etc.)	Additive or synergistic CNS depressant effect with acute ingestion of alcohol may occur	Mechanism: inhibition of hepatic metabolic enzymes Avoid concomitant use, esp. in patients with alcoholic liver disease Unpredictable tolerance may occur with chronic alcohol use Slight interaction occurs with use of small doses of ethanol, BZD, or both agents	Yes
Fluoxetine (Prozac)-diazepam	May enhance pharmacologic effects of diazepam	Fluoxetine may inhibit hepatic metabolism of diazepam	

		No specific precaution appears necessary	
Isoniazid–diazepam, triazolam	May ↑ actions of certain BZDs	Isoniazid may inhibit oxidative hepatic metabolism of BZD	?
Ketoconazole (Nizoral)-chloridiazepoxide	May ↓ clearance of chlordiazepoxide	Ketoconazole may inhibit some phase of liver degradation of chlordiazepoxide (?)	?
Levodopa–diazepam, chlordiazepoxide	Marked reduction in antiparkinsonian effect	Mechanism ? Consider discontinuing BZD if problem arises It is not known whether other BZDs would evoke a similar interaction	Yes
Lidocaine-diazepam	Enhances antiarrhythmic effect of lidocaine; protects against lidocaine-induced seizures (animal studies)	Mechanism ? No special precautions appear necessary	?
Lithium-diazepam	Hypothermia	Mechanism ? A single case report with several episodes of hypothermia during coadministration (idiosyncratic reaction?) No clinical interventions appear necessary	?

(Continued.)

Table 4–1 (cont.).

Combination	Interaction Effects	Mechanism/ Comment	Clinical Significance
Loxapine (Loxitane)-lorazepam	May ↑ pharmacologic or toxic effects of certan BZDs (CNS depression)	Mechanism ? Case reports proposed interaction Monitor vital signs during coadministration	?
Macrolide antibacterials (e.g., erythromycin, troleandomycin) triazolam	May ↑ CNS depression	Mechanism? Macrolide antibiotics are believed to inhibit hepatic metabolism of triazolam (other BZDs metabolized by oxidation?) No special precautions necessary	?
Muscle relaxants, nondepolarizing group (e.g., atracurium, gallamine triethiodide, pancuronium, tubocurarine, vecuronium) with diazepam, lorazepam, oxazepam	BZD may potentiate, counteract, or have no effect on actions of nondepolarizing muscle relaxants	Mechanism? Major problems have not been reported; be alert for any unusual effects	?
Omeprazole (Prilosec)-diazepam	May ↑ serum levels and pharmacologic effects of of diazepam	Omeprazole may inhibit oxidative hepatic metabolism of BZD During coadministration monitor clinical response to BZD and tailor dosage as needed	?

Phenytoin (Dilantin)–chlordiazepoxide, diazepam oxazepam	May ↑ serum phenytoin concentrations Phenytoin may ↑ oxazepam clearance	Mechanism ? Probably alteration of phenytoin metabolism Data conflicting Monitor phenytoin serum levels and effects when BZDs are added to or deleted from regimen	?
Probenecid (Benemid)–lorazepam, midazolam	A more rapid onset or more prolonged BZD effect may occur	Mechanism ? Probably probenecid interferenece with BZD conjugation in liver Be prepared for an earlier onset of BZD effect and observe for clinical signs of BZD accumulation during coadministration	?
Propofol (Diprivan)-diazepam	May ↑ pharmacologic effects of of propofol (e.g., excessive sedation)	Mechanism ? No special precautions appear necessary	?
Propranolol-diazepam	↑ Plasma diazepam levels	↓ Metabolism	?
Ranitidine (Zantac)-diazepam	May impair therapeutic actions of certain BZDs	Ranitidine may ↓ GI absorption of certain BZDs	Yes

(Continued.)

Table 4–1 (cont.).

Combination	Interaction Effects	Mechanism/ Comment	Clinical Significance
		Staggering administration may avoid interaction	
Rifampin (Rifadin)-diazepam	Increases clearance of diazepam and its metabolites (↓ diazepam effect)	Rifampin may stimulate oxidative metabolism Adjust the dose of diazepam during and after the coadministration	?
Smoking with chlordiazepoxide, diazepam, lorazepam	May ↓ BZD effect	Smoking may enhance hepatic metabolism of certain BZDs	?
Succinylcholine (Anectine) with diazepam, oxazepam	May antagonize, potentiate, or have no effect on actions of succinylcholine	Mechanism ? No special precautions appear necessary	?
Theophylines (aminophyline, theophyline)-diazepam	May ↓ sedative effects of diazepam	Mechanism ? Probably an antagonistic action by competitive binding to intracerebral adenosine receptor No special precautions appear necessary	Yes

Thyroid hormone–diazepam	May temporarily increase free (active) thyroxine levels	Diazepam displaces thryroxine and triiodothyronine from plasma protein binding Use this combination with caution	?
Valproate-diazepam	May ↑ pharmacokinetic parameters of diazepam	Valproate may inhibit diazepam oxidative metabolism; competitive inhibition of serum protein binding may also be responsible No clinical interventions appear necessary	

Clonazepam, flurazepam, halazepam, and prazepam may also be affected by cimetidine, etc. However, estrogens, cigarettes, xanthines (coffee), and rifampin, which induce microsomal enzymes, may reduce the therapeutic activity of the benzodiazepines that undergo oxidative metabolism. Benzodiazepines may react with some anticonvulsants and alter their metabolism; for example, benzodiazepines may affect the metabolism of carbamazepine and increase the rate of metabolism of clonazepam.

Triazolam and perhaps other benzodiazepines may be effected by coadministration of erythromycin which may produce an increase in serum concentrations of triazolam. This is due to an impairment in clearance.

Diazepam may reduce the renal excretion of digoxin, leading to possible digoxin toxicity. This may be true for other benzodiazepines as well. The interactions between benzodiazepines and tricyclic antidepressants (TCAs) are discussed in Chapter 1. Individual compounds within the benzodiazepine family may produce widely different abilities to cause adverse effects when coadministered with other medications. Hence, generalizations about benzodiazepine interactions do not apply to all drugs in this class. Attention must be paid to the specific benzodiazepine involved in any case report, or animal or human study. Table 4–1 reviews some of the interactions between benzodiazepines and other drugs.

Dosage and Administration

Dosage. The individual response to benzodiazepines varies widely, and for this reason individual dosages should be titrated to individual needs and tolerance. The lowest effective dose should be used. Caution should be exercised in administering this group of drugs to elderly or debilitated patients who may be more likely to develop significant side effects, especially confusion. In many cases, periodic readjustments of drug dosage may be required. Furthermore, the addition or removal of other drugs during benzodiazepine treatment may affect benzodiazepine concentrations. During prolonged administration, the need for benzodiazepines and their efficacy should be periodically reassessed. In patients with hepatic or renal disease, caution should be exercised, and the lowest possible effective dose should be used. In most cases, this will be 50% to 90% less than the dose used in otherwise healthy individuals.

Administration. In most cases, benzodiazepines are administered orally. Chlordiazepoxide and diazepam may also be administered intravenously (IV). Lorazepam may also be administered by IM injection. Erratic absorption precludes the IM administration of other benzodiazepines.

ALPRAZOLAM

Uses

Alprazolam is used most commonly for the treatment of anxiety disorders or short-term anxiety symptoms. It may also be helpful in the treatment of anxiety associated with depressive disorders. Recently, alprazolam also received Food and Drug Administration (FDA) approval for the treatment of panic disorder. The efficacy of alprazolam treatment in the control of anxiety symptoms has not been established for drug treatment which exceeds 4 months' of duration. As with all benzodiazepines, with prolonged administration, there should be periodic reassessments of drug efficacy and indications for treatment.

Cautions

Alprazolam shares many of the toxic effects of other benzodiazepines. (See the General Statement above for further details.) Like all benzodiazepines, alprazolam may produce withdrawal symptoms when abruptly discontinued. These may occur between 18 hours and 3 days after abrupt discontinuation of alprazolam. It is usually necessary that the patient be taking the drug for a period between 1 week and 4 months for withdrawal reactions to occur. The drug should be discontinued gradually in order to avoid abrupt withdrawal reactions.

The safety and efficacy of alprazolam has not been established in children younger than 18 years of age.

Dosage and Administration

Dosage. Alprazolam is given in divided doses. As with all benzodiazepines, dosage should be titrated to the individual's needs and tolerance, with the lowest effective dose being provided. In most cases the initial adult dosage is 0.25 to 0.5 mg three times a day; rarely is it necessary to exceed 4 mg/day. However, for the treatment of panic disorder, higher doses of 3 to 8 mg/day are usually necessary. If adverse side effects occur, the dosage should be reduced.

Administration. Alprazolam is administered orally.

Preparations

Alprazolam (*Xanax*)
Oral tablets
0.25 mg, 0.5 mg, 1.0 mg, 2.0 mg

CHLORDIAZEPOXIDE

Uses

Chlordiazepoxide is most commonly prescribed for the management of anxiety disorders or for the relief of anxiety symptoms. It is also commonly used for the management of acute alcohol withdrawal and its associated agitation. The efficacy of sustained administration of chlordiazepoxide beyond 4 months has not been established. Caution should be exercised when this drug is prescribed for a prolonged period of time. There should be periodic reassessments made of the continued need for therapy and continued responsiveness to drug treatment.

Dosage and Administration

Dosage. Dosage should be titrated to the individual's needs and tolerance, with the lowest effective dose being administered. Because chlordiazepoxide has a long half-life, as do its metabolites, care should be exercised when making dose adjustments. Although initially the drug is usually administered three or four times a day, after dosage has been stabilized most patients can be effectively managed with one or two doses each day. For the treatment of anxiety the usual dose is 5 to 10 mg three to four times a day. For severe anxiety the dose is 20 to 25 mg three or four times a day. For the management of anxiety associated with acute alcohol withdrawal the initial dose is 50 to 100 mg. Doses are repeated until agitation is controlled, with the daily dosage not exceeding 300 mg. The drug is gradually withdrawn over a 1- to 2-week period after alcohol withdrawal has been controlled.

In the geriatric population, in debilitated patients, and in children younger than 6 years of age, the initial dose should be 5 mg orally two to four times a day adjusted as necessary based on response. In children, this dosage may be increased to 10 mg two to three times a day. IV dosages are usually 50 to 100 mg as an initial bolus, followed by 25 to 50 mg three to four times a day as needed for adults. In the management of alcohol withdrawal–related anxiety the initial dose is usually 50 to 100 mg repeated every 2 to 4 hours, as needed. The parenteral dose should not exceed 300 mg in a 6-hour or 24-hour period.

Administration. Chlordiazepoxide is usually administered orally. It may also be administered by slow IV bolus in adults. Absorption following IM administration is erratic and for this reason this route should not be used.

Preparations

Chlordiazepoxide
  Oral tablets (*Libritabs*)
    5 mg, 10 mg, 25 mg
Chlordiazepoxide hydrochloride
  Oral capsules
    5 mg (*Librium*), 10 mg,
    (*Librium Mitran Resposans-10, Sereen*), 25 mg (*Librium*)
  Parenteral injection (*Librium*)
    100 mg

CLORAZEPATE DIPOTASSIUM

Uses

Clorazepate dipotassium is used in the management of anxiety disorder, anxiety symptoms, and in the treatment of anxiety and agitation associated with alcohol withdrawal. Clorazepate is also used adjunctively in the treatment of partial seizures. As with other benzodiazepines, the continued effectiveness of clorazepate dipotassium in prolonged administration beyond 4 months has not been fully documented. There should be ongoing assessment of the clinical indications and efficacy of this drug with prolonged treatment.

Cautions

Clorazepate dipotassium shares the toxic potentials of other benzodiazepines. (See the General Statement regarding benzodiazepines for complete details.)

Dosage and Administration

Dosage. Dosage of clorazepate dipotassium must be titrated to the individual's need and tolerance using the lowest effective dose. Dosage should be reduced in elderly and debilitated patients and in those with significant hepatic or renal disease. Clorazepate and its metabolites have half-lives which range up to 200 hours; this should be considered in making adjustments in dosage. In the treatment of anxiety, the usual initial dose is 30 mg/day given in divided doses. Once the patient has been stabilized the entire dose may be given at bedtime. Dosage adjustments should be made in gradual amounts. Rarely is it necessary to exceed 60 mg/day. In elderly, debilitated, or otherwise compromised patients, the usual initial dose may range from 7.5 to 15 mg/day given in divided doses.

For the treatment of acute alcohol withdrawal–associated anxiety the initial dose is 30 mg; this is followed by 30 to 60 mg in divided doses on the first day with the maximum not exceeding 90 mg/day. Subsequent dosage is adjusted as indicated by the clinical status.

Administration. Clorazepate dipotassium is administered orally. The 11.25- and 22.5-mg SD tablets may be used after patients have been stabilized on conventional tablets.

Preparations

Clorazepate dipotassium
- Oral capsules (*Clorazecaps*)
  - 3.75 mg, 7.5 mg, 15 mg
- Tablets
  - 3.75 mg, 7.5 mg (*Clorazetabs, Gene-XENE, Tranxene T-TAB*), 11.25 mg (*Tranxene-SD*), 15 mg (*Clorazetabs, Gene-XENE, Tranxene*), 22.5 mg (*Tranxene-SD*)

DIAZEPAM

Uses

Diazepam is used to control general symptoms of anxiety. Diazepam is also used in the treatment of agitation and other symptoms associated with acute alcohol withdrawal. The efficacy of diazepam during long term use of greater than 4 months' duration has not been established. For this reason care should be exercised with prolonged administration of diazepam. There should be periodic reassessments of the indications for continued drug treatment and drug efficacy.

Diazepam may be used to prevent night terrors by suppressing stage 4 sleep.

Cautions

Diazepam shares much of the side effect profile of other benzodiazepines. (See the General Statement regarding benzodiazepines for details.)

Care should be exercised when diazepam is administered parenterally. Rapid IV administration at a rate which exceeds 5 mg/min may produce hypotension or respiratory depression.

Dosage and Administration

Dosage. Dosage must be titrated to the individual's needs and tolerance. In general, the lowest clinically effective dose should be administered. Lower doses should be administered to elderly, debilitated patients, and to children. Diazepam and its metabolites have half lives which range from 20 to 100 hours. This should be considered when adjustments in dosage are undertaken.

Oral Dosage. The usual adult oral dosage of diazepam for the treatment of anxiety symptoms is 2 to 10 mg, two to four times per day. When extended capsules are used, 15 to 30 mg should be given once daily. For the treatment of agitation and anxiety associated with acute alcohol withdrawal, the usual dosage of oral diazepam is 10 mg three to four times a day during the first 24 hours. During subsequent days, dosage is usually 5 mg, three to four times a day as needed. For moderate to severe withdrawal reactions, 20 mg of diazepam may be needed every 1 to 2 hours until the symptoms are controlled. In patients with delirium tremens, an IV dose of 10 mg, followed by 5 mg every 5 minutes, may be necessary. Usually sedation and control is achieved within 30 minutes. Subsequent dosage requires titration via close observation to control symptoms, but with gradual withdrawal over the next 1 to 2 weeks. The treatment of night terrors in adults requires 5 to 20 mg of diazepam administered at bedtime.

In geriatric or debilitated patients, the usual initial dosage for anxiety symptoms is 2 mg twice a day or less. In children older than 6 months of age, the initial oral dosage is 1.0 to 2.5 mg, three or four times a day, as either an oral solution or as conventional tablets. Many clinicians use 0.12 to 0.8 mg/kg, in three or four divided doses, in children. The dosage is adjusted as needed and tolerated. The usual IV dose for moderate anxiety is 2.5 mg. For acute anxiety of a severe nature, it is 5 to 10 mg.

In general, dosages do not exceed 30 mg during an 8-hour period.

Administration. Diazepam is administered orally either as tablets or as an oral solution. It may also be administered by slow IV bolus at a rate which does not exceed 5 mg/min in adults. After stable serum levels have been achieved the drug may be administered orally one or two times per day. During IV administration, the drug should be administered only into large veins to avoid thrombosis. Administration into small veins, arteries, or extravasation may produce tissue damage. IM absorption is erratic; therefore, this route is not preferred.

Preparations

Diazepam
- Oral capsules, extended-release (*Valrelease*)
  - 15 mg
- Solution (*Diazepam Solution*)
  - 5 mg/5 mL
- Solution, concentrate (*Diazepam Intensol*)
  - 5 mg/mL
- Tablets (*Q-pam, Valium*)
  - 2 mg, 5 mg, 10 mg
- Parenteral (*T-Quil, Valium, Zetran*)
  - Injection 5 mg/mL

FLURAZEPAM HYDROCHLORIDE

Uses

Flurazepam is used for the short-term treatment of insomnia for up to 4 weeks. It shares the other actions of benzodiazepines. As with all benzodiazepines continued indications for use and continued documentation of efficacy should be assessed with prolonged administration.

Cautions

Flurazepam shares the side effect profile of other benzodiazepines. (Consult the General Statement regarding benzodiazepines for complete details.)

Dosage and Administration

Dosage. Dosage should be individualized to the patient's needs and tolerance with lower dosages being given to elderly and debilitated patients. In general, the lowest clinically effective dose should be prescribed. In most adults, the usual hypnotic dose is 30 mg at bedtime; 15 mg may be effective in many patients. In debilitated or geriatric patients the initial dose should be 15 mg.

Administration. Flurazepam is administered orally.

Preparations

Flurazepam hydrochloride (*Dalmane*)
  Oral capsules
    15 mg, 30 mg

HALAZEPAM

Uses

Halazepam shares the therapeutic actions of other benzodiazepines. It is usually supplied to patients for the treatment of anxiety symptoms or the treatment of anxiety disorders. As with all benzodiazepines, the efficacy of administration of halazepam beyond 4 months has not been established. Continued reassessment of indications and effectiveness should be undertaken with prolonged drug treatment.

Cautions

See the General Statement regarding benzodiazepines. In general, halazepam shares the side effect profile of other benzodiazepines.

Dosage and Administration

Dosage. Dosage should be individualized to the patient's needs and tolerance using the smallest clinically effective dose. The usual initial adult oral dosage is 20 to 40 mg, three to four times a day. Dosage is then adjusted in response to the needs of the patient, usually to between 80 and 160 mg/day. In the elderly or in debilitated patients, the usual initial dosage is 20 mg, once or twice a day.

Administration. Halazepam is administered orally in divided doses.

Preparations

Halazepam
  Oral tablets (*Paxipam*)
    20 mg, 40 mg

LORAZEPAM

Uses

Lorazepam is indicated in the management of symptoms of anxiety disorders or for the relief of anxiety symptoms associated with depressive conditions. It shares the general actions of the benzodiazepines. As with all benzodiazepines, the need for continued treatment should be periodically reassessed as should drug efficacy. The effectiveness of lorazepam in long-term treatment (greater than 4 months) has not been established.

Cautions

See the General Statement regarding benzodiazepines for complete details. Caution should be exercised when CNS depressant drugs are coadministered with benzodiazepines such as lorazepam because of the possibility of an additive effect. Such drugs include the phenothiazines, opiate agonists, antidepressants, alcohol, and barbiturates. When used in high dosages, or with other CNS depressants, care should be exercised to prevent respiratory depression. This is especially problematic in elderly or debilitated patients, who in general should receive lower doses than young healthy adults. Likewise, patients with renal or hepatic failure may be more sensitive to drug effects since lorazepam is conjugated in the liver and excreted via the kidneys. In these patients, the lowest possible effective dose should be used. As with all benzodiazepines, lorazepam may impair the patient's ability to operate hazardous machinery or engage in other activities which require mental alertness or physical coordination. Patients should be educated regarding this effect prior to drug administration. These effects may be potentiated by the coadministration of other CNS depressant drugs and may be of extended duration in elderly, debilitated patients, or patients with hepatic or renal disease. Lorazepam should be used with caution in the oral form in children younger than 18 years of age; the drug has not been established as safe and efficacious in children under the age of 12 years when administered as an injection.

Mutagenicity and Carcinogenicity. There is no evidence of carcinogenicity in animal studies. Research studies to evaluate mutagenicity have not been performed.

Pregnancy, Fertility, and Lactation. Care should be exercised when lorazepam is administered to pregnant women, since it may produce fetal toxicity. In particular, congenital malformation may be associated with the early administration of these agents. The drug is known to cross the placenta; therefore it is not only contraindicated during pregnancy but is contraindicated during active labor and delivery. Patients should be cautioned about becoming pregnant while taking lorazepam. It is unknown if lorazepam is distributed into human breast milk. However, other benzodiazepines are found in human breast milk, and for this reason caution should be used in the administration of lorazepam to nursing women.

Lorazepam is not known to affect fertility in humans. There is no evidence of impaired fertility in rodents.

Dosage and Administration

Dosage.. Dosage should be titrated to the individual's needs and tolerance. The lowest clinically effective dose should be administered. In the treatment of anxiety, the usual initial dosage is 2 to 3 mg/day, in two or three divided doses. In the elderly or debilitated patient, the usual initial dosage is 1 to 2 mg/day in divided dosages. It is rarely advisable for total daily dosage to exceed 10 mg/day in divided doses.

Administration. Lorazepam is administered orally as tablets or by IM or IV injection.

Preparations

Lorazepam
- Oral tablets (*Ativan, Loraz*)
  - 0.5 mg, 1.0 mg, 2.0 mg
- Parenteral injection (*Ativan*)
  - 2 mg/mL, 4 mg/mL

OXAZEPAM

Uses

Oxazepam shares the clinical effectiveness of other benzodiazepines and is used predominantly in the management of insomnia or anxiety symptoms, either as a part of an anxiety disorder or associated with depressive syndromes. It is also useful in the short-term treatment of insomnia, anxiety, agitation, and other symptoms associated with acute alcohol withdrawal.

Cautions

Oxazepam shares the toxic potential of other benzodiazepines. (See the General Statement regarding benzodiazepines for details.) The safety and efficacy of oxazepam have not been established for patients younger than 6 years of age.

Dosage and Administration

Dosage. Dosage should be titrated to the individual's needs and tolerance, and the smallest clinically effective dose administered. In most cases the usual initial dose for the treatment of anxiety is 10 to 15 mg three to four times a day. For severe anxiety or in treating anxiety associated with acute alcohol withdrawal, 15 to 30 mg may be given three to four times a day. In elderly and debilitated patients, 10 mg three times a day is the usual initial dosage.

Administration. Oxazepam is administered orally.

Preparations

Oxazepam
- Oral capsules (*Serax, Zaxopram*)
  - 10 mg, 15 mg, 30 mg
- Tablets (*Serax*)
  - 15 mg

PRAZEPAM

Uses

Prazepam shares the actions of other benzodiazepines. (See the General Statement regarding benzodiazepines for complete details.) In brief, prazepam is effective for the treatment of anxiety associated with anxiety disorders or with depressive syndromes.

Cautions

Prazepam shares the toxic potentials of other benzodiazepines. (See the General Statement regarding benzodiazepines for complete details.) In particular, caution should be exercised in the administration of this drug to patients who may engage in driving, operating machinery, or other hazardous activities. Patients should be informed about the possible risks of engaging in such activities.

Dosage and Administration

Dosage. Dosage should be titrated to the individual's need and tolerance, with the lowest clinically effective dose provided.

Prazepam and its metabolites have half-lives extending to approximately 200 hours; this should be considered when making dosage adjustments. In general, the initial dosage in most patients is 30 mg/day, in divided doses. Ultimately, this may range up to 60 mg/day. After initial stabilization, the drug may be administered as one single dose at bedtime. In debilitated and elderly patients, the usual initial dosages are 10 to 15 mg/day, in divided doses.

Administration. Prazepam is administered orally.

Preparations

Prazepam (*Centrax*)
  Oral
    Capsules: 5 mg, 10 mg, 20 mg
    Tablets: 10 mg

QUAZEPAM

Uses

Quazepam is reported to be selective for one of the two types of benzodiazepine (BZ) receptors, i.e., the BZ-1 receptor. The clinical effect and importance of this selectivity has not been established, but in theory this benzodiazepine may be less likely to cause changes in cognitive or motor functioning. So far, studies have not shown the development of drug tolerance during the first 4 weeks of use. In addition, initial studies show no rebound insomnia following 4 weeks of use at a dose of 15 mg per night. The most frequent side effect of quazepam is daytime drowsiness. The clinical efficacy of quazepam has not been established for use longer than 4 weeks.

Cautions

Until the clinical effect of receptor selectivity becomes clear, it is probably best to observe the same cautions regarding Quazepam use as for other benzodiazepines. (See the General Statement regarding benzodiazepines for complete details.) Specifically, caution should be exercised in the administration of this drug to patients who may engage in driving, operating machinery, or other hazardous activities. Patients should be informed about the possible risks of engaging in such activities, and that impairment of performance may extend to the day following medication use.

Dosage and Administration

Dosage. The dose of quazepam should be titrated to the individual's need and tolerance. The lowest clinically effective dose should be used. Quazepam and its metabolites have half-lives that may extend for more than 150 hours. This should be taken into consideration when adjusting dosage; this is especially critical in debilitated or elderly patients, who may clear the drug even more slowly. The initial dose is usually 15 mg at bedtime; after a few days, this can often be reduced to 7.5 mg. For elderly or debilitated patients, it may be best to start with a dose of 7.5 mg.

Administration. Quazepam is administered orally.

Preparations

Quazepam (*Doral*)
  Oral tablets
    7.5 mg, 15 mg

TEMAZEPAM

Uses

Temazepam shares the clinical actions of other benzodiazepines. (See the General Statement regarding benzodiazepines for complete details.) In brief, the drug is an effective hypnotic for the short-term relief of insomnia. Its clinical efficacy has not been established for treatment periods longer than 5 weeks' duration. If patients are treated for longer periods of time the drug should be assessed for continued efficacy and the indications for continuing treatment should be reassessed.

Cautions

Temazepam shares the toxic potentials of other benzodiazepines. (See the General Statement regarding benzodiazepines for complete details.) Specifically, however, the safety and efficacy of temazepam has not been established in persons younger than 18 years of age. Furthermore, patients should be cautioned about engaging in activities such as driving vehicles or operating machinery while under the influence of temazepam.

Dosage and Administration

Dosage. Dosage should be individualized to the patient's needs and tolerance, with the lowest clinically effective dose provided. Lower dosages should be used in the elderly and in debilitated patients. The usual initial oral dosage is 30 mg/day. In many patients, in particular the elderly and debilitated, 15 mg may be adequate.

Administration Temazepam is administered orally.

Preparations

Temazepam (*Restoril, Temaz*)
  Oral capsules
    15 mg, 30 mg

TRIAZOLAM

Uses

Triazolam shares the actions of other benzodiazepines. (See the General Statement regarding benzodiazepines for complete details.) In general, triazolam is used in the treatment of insomnia. Its efficacy has not been established for continuous treatment beyond 6 weeks' duration. In such cases, the drug should be assessed for continued efficacy as a hypnotic and the clinical indications should also be reassessed. Triazolam has a very short half-life; therefore, it is more appropriate for the treatment of initial insomnia, i.e., difficulty in falling asleep, than for mid- or early awakening.

Cautions

Triazolam shares the toxic potential of other benzodiazepines. (See the General Statement regarding benzodiazepines for complete details.) In general, however, patients should be cautioned about engaging in hazardous activities such as operating machinery or driving motor vehicles when under the influence of triazolam. The safety and efficacy of triazolam has not been established in persons younger than 18 years of age.

Dosage and Administration

Dosage. Dosage should be titrated to the individual's needs and tolerance, with the lowest clinically effective dose provided. The dosage should be reduced in elderly or debilitated patients. The usual initial dosage is 0.25 mg; for many patients, in particular the elderly and debilitated, 0.125 mg may be adequate. Occasionally some patients may require a dose of 0.5 mg.

Administration. Triazolam is administered orally.

Preparations

Triazolam (*Halcion*)
  Oral tablets
    0.125 mg, 0.25 mg

ANTIPSYCHOTICS 5

GENERAL STATEMENT

Antipsychotic drugs, a chemically diverse class of drugs, share many pharmacologic properties, which warrants their discussion within a single chapter. While at times they are referred to as major tranquilizers, antischizophrenic drugs, and neuroleptics, such labeling of the antipsychotic medications is unwarranted. Tranquilization (sedation) is not necessary for therapeutic effect; the antipsychotics vary greatly in their ability to produce tranquilization; many tranquilizing medications are without antipsychotic effect; and tolerance usually develops to the tranquilizing effects of the antipsychotics but not to the antipsychotic effects. While the antipsychotics are now the principle agents used in the treatment of schizophrenia, they are also used in other nonschizophrenic psychoses.

The term *neuroleptics* is the term most often substituted for antipsychotic agents, primarily for historical reasons. The antipsychotic medications were referred to as neuroleptics because of their ability to produce the neuroleptic syndrome. This syndrome consists of decreased spontaneous motor activity, depressed initiative, decreased affect, disinterest in surroundings, and suppression of complex behavior. In the late 1940s and early 1950s the early research on phenothiazines (PTZs) focused on this ability to diminish arousal as a method for potentiating anesthesia. Subsequently it became clear that these drugs were useful in the treatment of agitated psychotic patients, but it was initially believed that neurolepsis was necessary for their antipsychotic effects. It has since been recognized, however, that neurolepsis is a side effect of many of these agents, not correlating with the therapeutic effect. These neuroleptic effects are now recognized as unnecessary, unpleasant, and a common cause of discontinuation of the medications by the patients. Furthermore, the newest antipsychotic, clozapine, is an extremely effective drug that does not appear to cause neurolepsis. The best-established indication for antipsychotics is in the treatment of schizophrenia. These agents have proved quite effective in suppressing the hallucinations, thought disorder, and delusions of schizophrenia. They also appear to be effective in the treatment of psychotic symptoms in other disorders such as organic psychoses, mood disorders with psychotic features, paranoid disorder, schizophreniform disorder, brief reactive psychosis, atypical psychosis, and schizoaffective disorder.

While the focus of this chapter is on the use of antipsychotics in the treatment of psychiatric disorders, it should also be recognized that there are a variety of nonpsychiatric uses for these medications including nausea and vomiting, intractable hiccups, chronic pain, some movement disorders, and they continue to be used as an adjunct to anesthetic agents.

There are six classes of antipsychotics currently available in the United States: the PTZs, thioxanthenes, butyrophenones, dibenzoxazepines, dihydroindolones, and, most recently, the dibenzodiazepines. There is a seventh class, the diphenylbutylpiperidines; however, pimozide (Orap), the only representative of this class in the United States, is primarily used in the treatment of Gilles de la Tourette's syndrome, though it does have antipsychotic properties. While these six classes of compounds have very different chemistries, their pharmacologic effects are quite similar, varying only in potency (the dibenzodiazepines may be an exception). While the severity of the side effects induced may vary among the individual classes, no single antipsychotic has ever been proved more effective than any other, except, perhaps, the newly released dibenzodiazepine, clozapine.

The PTZs constitute the prototypal class of antipsychotic and thus this introductory section of the chapter will describe the general features of PTZs. The second section will describe the individual antipsychotics.

EFFECTS

Behavioral. Initiative and interest in the environment are reduced after neuroleptic administration. The display of emotions is also diminished, and in animals the usual highly reinforcing electrical self-stimulation of the medial forebrain bundle is blocked. The PTZs block dopaminergic agonist-induced emesis, presumably by blockade of dopamine receptor in the medullary chemoreceptor trigger zone. The hyperactivity and aggressiveness that is induced by the dopaminergic agonists is also blocked.

Motor Activity. The PTZs all reduce spontaneous motor activity. In high doses they can cause rigidity that resembles the catatonia seen in some psychotic patients. The PTZs often produce extrapyramidal effects, including parkinsonism, dystonia, akathisia, and tardive dyskinesia. The parkinsonism may be complete with bradykinesia, akinesia, cogwheel rigidity, masked facies, stooped posture, and shuffling gait. Akathisia is characterized by a highly unpleasant inner sense of restlessness which often motivates the individual taking PTZs to pace ceaselessly owing to a subjective sense of being unable to sit still. It can be very difficult to distinguish this side effect from psychotic agitation.

Nervous System. The PTZs block dopamine receptors throughout the central nervous system (CNS) with little effect on spinal reflexes. Dopamine blockade in specific brain regions probably accounts for many of the untoward effects of these agents and may account for the therapeutic effect.

The antipsychotic effects of PTZs may be due to their ability to block dopaminergic pathways between the midbrain and limbic system (the mesolimbic pathways) and the pathways between the midbrain and the frontal and temporal cortices (the mesocortical pathways). The parkinsonian-like side effects of the PTZs are thought to be due to their dopamine blocking activity in the nigrostriatal pathway (from the substantia nigra to the caudate head).

The tuberoinfundibular system projecting from the arcuate nucleus of the hypothalamus to the median eminence is also a dopamine-rich pathway affected by PTZs. The release of prolactin from the pituitary is blocked by the effect of dopamine in the tuberoinfundibular system. Thus, PTZs enhance prolactin secretion (and elevate serum prolactin levels) by blocking the dopamine neurons of this system. While tolerance appears to develop to the dopamine blocking effects of PTZs in the nigrostriatal pathway and tuberoinfundibular system, the mesolimbic and mesocortical areas do not become tolerant to the dopamine blocking effects.

The antidopaminergic properties of PTZs also appear to account for their ability to block the nausea and emesis-inducing effects of apomorphine, which acts as an agonist on central dopaminergic receptors, including the chemoreceptor trigger zone of the medulla.

All effective antipsychotics appear to mediate some depression of vasomotor reflexes in the hypothalamus or brainstem, presumably resulting in a centrally mediated hypotension. However, from a clinical standpoint these effects are minimal and rarely cause clinically significant drops in blood pressure. There is very little effect of the PTZs on the respiratory centers of the brainstem and thus in most cases they have virtually no effect on respiration.

In humans, the PTZs produce a slowing of the electroencephalogram (EEG) with an increase in theta and delta waves. There is a mild decrease in alpha waves and fast beta activity accompanying an increase in spike activity. Thus the PTZs, and in particular the aliphatic subclass, can lower the seizure threshold, though usually this is clinically irrelevant except in patients with family or personal histories of seizure disorders or patients undergoing alcohol or sedative withdrawal. Though controversial, some experts consider fluphenazine and molindone to be the least epileptogenic neuroleptics.

The PTZs block α_1-adrenergic receptors in the autonomic ganglia which presumably accounts for most of their ability to produce postural hypotension, and may account for the inhibition of ejaculation which can occur, especially with thioridazine. Furthermore, like heterocyclic antidepressants, the PTZs and other antipsychotics are capable of blocking muscarinic receptors. Though they are less potent than the heterocyclic antidepressants at blocking muscarinic receptors, they can produce clinically important anticholinergic side effects. These may include blurred vision, constipation, decreased sweating, dryness of mucous membranes, and, rarely, urinary retention. Finally, the PTZs also appear to block serotonin and histamine receptors, which may account for some of their sedating and appetite-increasing effects in animals and humans.

Cardiovascular. The effects of the PTZs on the cardiovascular system are complex since they produce direct effects on the heart and blood vessels, and indirectly affect the cardiovascular system through their actions in the nervous system. The most common cardiovascular effect is postural hypotension with reflex tachycardia. This is secondary to the peripheral and central α-adrenergic blockade produced by PTZs. The PTZs, apparently owing to their structural similarity to quinidine, have some antiarrhythmic effect and can prolong QT and PR intervals with blunting of T waves. PTZs (especially thioridazine) can produce ventricular arrhythmias and sudden death.

Hepatic. Rarely, hypersensitivity reactions associated with the use of PTZs have been reported, occasionally producing an elevation of serum liver enzymes, consistent with obstructive jaundice. These drugs can be used in patients with hepatic disease, though careful monitoring is indicated since their metabolism can be altered in the presence of liver damage.

Endocrine. As described above, the PTZs can increase prolactin secretion with subsequent development of amenorrhea and galactorrhea in women. Gynecomastia may occur in men. Growth hormone secretion is diminished and secretion of adrenocortical steroids may also be suppressed.

Hematologic. PTZs are occasionally associated with mild and usually transient depression of leukopoiesis. Rarely—in about 1 case in 10,000—agranulocytosis may occur. The mortality is high; therefore, fever, sore throat, or cellulitis are indications for stopping the drug and obtaining a complete blood count (CBC) with differential. This risk is much higher with clozapine, occurring in up to 1% to 2% of patients.

Dermatologic. Allergic reactions with urticarial, maculopapular, or petechial lesions occur infrequently, and there have been occasional reports of exfoliative dermatitis. Photosensitivity may occur in the form of acute, severe sunburn or rash, or chronic purplish-brown pigmentation.

Pharmacokinetics

Absorption. Orally administered PTZs are erratically and variably absorbed from the gastrointestinal (GI) tract. Parenteral administration, however, can increase the availability of the PTZs by 4 to 10 times.

Distribution. These drugs are tightly bound to plasma protein and widely distributed in the body. They are highly lipophilic and thus accumulate in fat stores, readily cross the placenta to the fetus, and are secreted in breast milk.

Effects. The plasma half-lives of PTZs typically range from 10 to 20 hours though the biological effects after a single dose can last as long as 24 hours. When administered chronically, the lipid-rich tissues of the body, including the brain, slowly release the PTZs which are then metabolized in the liver. Most of the PTZs are oxidized by the hepatic microsomal enzymes. These hydrophilic metabolites are then excreted primarily in the urine and to a small extent in the bile. Many of the metabolites are biologically active and thus confound the correlation of plasma levels of the parent compound with clinical effects.

Uses

Psychiatric. Neuroleptic drugs are the principle treatment for schizophrenia. These drugs had a revolutionary effect on the treatment of schizophrenia since they were the first family of drugs useful for the specific symptoms of psychosis, unlike the formerly used sedatives.

The PTZs are also effective in the treatment of schizoaffective disorder, mood disorders with psychotic features, and for psychoses associated with organic brain disorders such as delirium.

The sedating effects of the PTZs are also helpful for treating agitated or explosive behavior in acute settings associated with psychotic disorders, severe behavioral disorders in children, or in certain neurodegenerative diseases, such as Alzheimer's.

Various neuropsychiatric disorders associated with movement disorders have also been treated successfully with neuroleptics, including Gilles de la Tourette's syndrome and Huntington's disease.

Nonpsychiatric. Phenothiazines are helpful for the prevention and control of nausea and vomiting. Certain phenothiazines such as chlorpromazine (CPZ) have also been used in the treatment of intractable hiccups. In addition, they are known to exert an antipruritic effect and may be helpful in relieving psychogenic itching, as well as aid in the treatment of neurodermatitis and eczema.

The PTZs are also used as an adjunct in the induction of anesthesia and for some chronic pain conditions.

Cautions

The PTZs produce a wide variety of side effects that are unfortunately fairly common, quite unpleasant, often a cause of discontinuation of the medication by the patient, and at times irreversible.

Extrapyramidal Symptoms. Persons receiving phenothiazines may develop extrapyramidal symptoms. These adverse effects appear to be due to the blockade of central dopaminergic receptors involved in motor function. They occur more commonly in high doses and can usually be relieved by reducing the dose. Extrapyramidal reactions can be subdivided into dystonic reactions, akathisia, parkinsonism, and tardive dyskinesia. Acute dystonic reactions producing facial grimacing, torticollis, and occasionally oculogyric crises can occur during early stages of treatment with a PTZ. Involuntary contractions of the neck, facial, jaw, and perioral musculature are common. Opisthotonos (neck spasms, arching the head backward) can also occur. Dystonic reactions can be painful to the patient and unpleasant for family members. The symptoms are episodic and, like most extrapyramidal symptoms, can be overcome voluntarily for brief periods. However, after maintaining the normal posture against a dystonic reaction, typically the patient tires and the body part "snaps back" into the dystonic posture. Though uncomfortable, dystonic reactions are rarely dangerous, though there have been some cases of respiratory distress associated with laryngeal and diaphragmatic reactions. Most often, the dystonic reactions occur within the first few days of therapy, or after an increase in the drug dosage.

Tetanus, seizures, conversion reactions, and hypocalcemia must be considered in the differential diagnosis of a dystonic reaction though accurate diagnosis of a dystonic reaction is usually not difficult if the history reveals that the patient has recently begun an antipsychotic drug, or increased the dose or potency of the antipsychotic. The higher-potency antipsychotics are most likely to produce acute dystonia and young males are at greatest risk. Treatment with antiparkinsonian agents such as benztropine, trihexyphenidyl, or diphenhydramine administered parenterally will usually produce a rapid reversal of the dystonic reaction. The clinician should keep in mind that these antiparkinsonian agents have a much shorter half-life than most neuroleptics; therefore, the patient is at risk for recurrence of the dystonic signs after the antiparkinsonian agent has been excreted.

Akathisia is a symptom characterized by a desire to remain in constant motion. The patient often describes feeling "nervous" or "jittery" and is often seen pacing the halls or marching in place. Akathisia may occur early in treatment, after chronic treatment, or after a single dose of a PTZ, such as might be used for the treatment of nausea in a nonpsychotic individual. The incidence has been reported to be up to 45% in some studies. The unpleasant nature of this symptom, which often goes unrecognized or misdiagnosed as anxiety or increased agitation, is reflected in the fact that it appears to be the most common cause of self-discontinuation of PTZs. There may or may not be overt motor manifestations and the drug may be associated only with the subjective sensation of restlessness. Anticholinergic agents, benzodiazepines, and propranolol have all been used with varying effect to reduce akathisia. At times, a lower neuroleptic dose or an alternative neuroleptic may reduce akathisia.

A parkinsonian syndrome with akinesia, masked facies, reduced spontaneous movement, rigidity, and a pill-rolling tremor is a common manifestation of a PTZ-induced extrapyramidal disorder. Shuffling gait with en bloc turning, drooling, and slow monotonous speech is also part of the picture. Geriatric patients and those with organic brain damage appear to be especially susceptible to the development of this parkinsonian syndrome. Like akathisia, anticholinergics and dosage reduction can ameliorate these symptoms, usually more successfully than for akathisia.

Tardive dyskinesia consists of involuntary aimless movements of the tongue, face, mouth, or jaw which may at times also involve other motor groups such as the extremities or diaphragm. This syndrome is associated with long-term administration of PTZs. The movements often include lip-smacking, chewing, and protrusion of the tongue. If the extremities are involved the patient will often display rapid, jerky choreiform movements or writhing athetoid movements, or both. The elderly are at highest risk for development of tardive dyskinesia. Some studies indicate that females, individuals with mood disorders, and patients with brain damage may be particularly prone to the development of tardive dyskinesia. Some patients are unaware of any of the abnormal movements. The dyskinesia is generally painless and can be voluntarily suppressed. Like other extrapyramidal disorders, tardive dyskinesia disappears during sleep. Estimates of the incidence of tardive dyskinesia range from 10% to 50% in patients who are treated with neuroleptics chronically. The optimal approach is prevention. PTZs should not be used to treat relatively benign conditions such as anxiety or nonpsychotic depression. When used, they should be prescribed in the lowest dose for the shortest time possible. Patients taking PTZs should undergo periodic routine screening for tardive dyskinesia. If movements are detected, discussion with the patient and his or her family about dosage reduction or medication discontinuation should be undertaken.

The differential diagnosis of tardive dyskinesia includes Huntington's disease, Wilson's disease, withdrawal dyskinesia (spontaneous emergence of a dyskinesia associated with reduction of phenothiazine dosage), and idiopathic dyskinesia. Though no specific treatments have been developed to reverse tardive dyskinesia, evidence is emerging that the side effect is not necessarily progressive nor even permanent in all patients, even those continued on PTZs.

Sedation. Though all PTZs cause sedation, the degree to which individual agents produce this side effect varies widely. Generally, the low-potency neuroleptics cause more sedation. Furthermore, tolerance develops to this effect usually after the first few weeks.

Seizures. Many PTZs can lower the seizure threshold and thus place patients with seizure disorders at increased risk for development of a seizure. The aliphatic PTZs with low potency seem particularly prone to produce epileptiform discharges. The high-potency PTZs, particularly piperazine and the thioxanthenes, and the dihydroindolone molindone, appear to have very little effect on seizure activity.

Neuroleptic Malignant Syndrome (NMS). This syndrome consists of autonomic instability, altered mental status, and fluctuating levels of consciousness which may progress to stupor, severe muscle hypertonicity, and hyperthermia. It can be induced by all neuroleptics, and is potentially life-threatening. Autonomic effects often include diaphoresis, fluctuations in blood pressure, pallor, and cardiac arrhythmias. There may be akinesia along with rigidity. The continued muscle hypertonicity produces an increase in serum creatine kinase (CK). This syndrome may progress to rhabdomyolysis with subsequent myoglobinuria which can produce renal failure. Leukocytosis may also occur.

NMS may occur at any point during the course of treatment with neuroleptics. Some patients who develop NMS have no difficulty with subsequent rechallenging with PTZs. Risk factors for NMS include heat stress, debilitation, physical exhaustion, and concurrent organic brain disease. Use of long-acting depot neuroleptic preparations may also be a risk factor.

In most cases, NMS progresses rapidly over 2 to 3 days after the initial manifestations. Death may occur from cardiac arrhythmias, cardiovascular collapse, aspiration pneumonia, rhabdomyolysis with renal failure, or respiratory failure. Treatment should include discontinuation of the PTZ, correction of fluid and electrolyte balances, general supportive care, and cooling of the patient. Dantrolene, bromocriptine, amantadine, and benzodiazepines have been used with varying success in the treatment of NMS.

PTZs may also produce hypothermia or heat stroke due to impairment of hypothalamic thermoregulatory mechanisms.

Anticholinergic Effects. The anticholinergic effects of the PTZs can produce blurred vision, dry mouth, urinary retention, decreased intestinal motility, and constipation, impotence, and increased heart rate. These side effects usually resolve within a few weeks as a result of the development of tolerance but can usually be managed by lowering the dose. Anticholinergic effects also tend to precipitate delirium, particularly in the elderly, or in patients with organic brain syndromes.

Cardiovascular Effects. Orthostatic hypotension due to α-adrenergic blockade is the most common cardiovascular complication of PTZ therapy. The elderly are at greater risk than younger patients. Tolerance usually develops to this effect. The PTZs can be antiarrhythmic or arrhythmogenic. The antiarrhythmic effects appear to be due to local lidocaine-like effects and quinidine-like effects on the myocardium and cardiac conduction system.

The arrhythmogenic effects appear to be related to their ability to prolong QT and PR intervals with T wave changes and depression of the ST segment. Thioridazine is the PTZ most often implicated as arrhythmogenic.

Cutaneous Effects. Patients may develop a skin photosensitivity and should be warned to avoid prolonged sun exposure and to use a sun screen.

Ophthalmologic Effects. Extended treatment with high doses of low-potency PTZs has been associated with retinal, corneal, conjunctival, and lens pigmentation. This effect is usually clinically insignificant though the pigmentary retinopathy associated with the prolonged use of thioridazine in doses above 800 mg/day can result in visual impairment. Thus, doses of thioridazine should be less than 800 mg/day.

Hematologic Effects. Hematologic effects may include agranulocytosis, mild leukopenia, and less commonly eosinophilia and aplastic anemia. The incidence of agranulocytosis with the low-potency neuroleptics has been estimated to be as high as 1 in 4,000. Thus, sore throat, fever, or other signs of infection should prompt the physician to obtain a white blood cell (WBC) count and differential. If the WBC count is low, the PTZ should be discontinued.

Fertility, Pregnancy, and Lactation. Because of their high lipophilicity, PTZs readily cross the placenta and are secreted in breast milk. Thus, PTZs should be used with caution in pregnant women. The butyrophenones appear to have little, if any, teratogenic effects. Lactating mothers should be advised not to breastfeed while taking PTZs.

Toxicity

Manifestations. Overdosage of PTZs tends to produce an exacerbation of the underlying common adverse effects. Severe extrapyramidal symptoms, sedation, and hypotension are most commonly reported. CNS depression may progress to areflexia with coma. Electrocardiographic (ECG) changes and tachyarrhythmias can occur. There may be hypothermia with an increased muscle tone, difficulty swallowing or breathing, and vasomotor collapse.

Treatment. Generally, treatment involves systemic and supportive care. Anticholinergic, antiparkinsonian agents may be helpful in reducing extrapyramidal symptoms, though caution is indicated regarding the anticholinergics, which might exacerbate underlying anticholinergic toxicity. After acute drug ingestion, the drug may be removed from the stomach by gastric lavage. Epinephrine should be avoided in the treatment of hypotension because PTZs may reverse the vasopressor effects of epinephrine and further lower blood pressure. Hemodialysis is usually not helpful.

Drug Interactions

The clinical interaction between antipsychotics and other drugs involves the levels of absorption and alterations in metabolism and receptor activity (Table 5–1). Two types of alteration in antipsychotic absorption have been reported. In the first, antacids may decrease the absorption of PTZs by forming a complex with them. The second is the anticholinergic effect on GI motility, and the slowed transit time enhancing metabolism of CPZ and other PTZs in the intestine. In addition to reducing GI motility, antipsychotics may enhance the absorption of other drugs, such as corticosteroids and digoxin.

Coadministration of PTZ and propranolol has been shown to cause a significant increase in plasma concentrations of both drugs, along with increased pharmacologic effect. In one study, the combination of propranolol and haloperidol failed to produce this finding. This implies that when propranolol is administered along with an antipsychotic agent to control violent or agitated behavior, it would be safer to use haloperidol rather than a PTZ. However, a case report documents the occurrence of hypotension and cardiopulmonary arrest with concurrent haloperidol and propranolol therapy. Both increased and decreased levels of phenytoin are reported with concomitant antipsychotic treatment. Because PTZ affects carbohydrate metabolism, the PTZ-induced increase in blood glucose levels may require alterations in insulin or oral hypoglycemic agent dosages in diabetics. The rate of antipsychotic metabolism is affected by a number of drugs that enhance or inhibit the cytochrome P-450 system. Drugs that enhance antipsychotic metabolism (decreased antipsychotic action) are barbiturates, nonbarbiturate hypnotics, carbamazepine, griseofulvin, phenylbutazone, and rifampin. Drugs that inhibit metabolism are acetaminophen, chloramphenicol, disulfiram, monoamine oxidase inhibitors (MAOIs), oral contraceptives, and the tricyclic antidepressants (TCAs).

Antipsychotics affect the receptor activity of many types of drugs. In the CNS, they counteract amphetamine toxicity and inhibit the appetite-depressing effect of amphetamine and the amphetamine-like compounds. The antiparkinsonian effects of levodopa can be reversed by antipsychotic agents, and levodopa itself may counter antipsychotic effects and exacerbate psychosis. In a parkinsonian patient who requires antipsychotic treatment, it may be best to utilize anticholinergic, antiparkinsonian agents alone or combined with amantadine to control symptoms of the movement disorder. The α-adrenergic blocking activity of PTZs can lead to significant hypotension when used in combination with coronary, cerebral, or peripheral vasodilators or with antihypertensive drugs. Likewise, the combination of a PTZ with an MAOI antidepressant may produce profound hypotension. Treatment of hypotension caused by these drug interactions with a mixed α- and β-agonist such as epinephrine can produce even more severe hypotension because of the unopposed β-agonist vasodilator activity.

Haloperidol (with the least α-adrenergic blocking effect) and the piperazine phenothiazines (e.g., trifluoperazine) are safer if used in conjunction with MAOIs than are the lower-potency, more hypotensive antipsychotics. Use of anesthetics such as halothane, enflurance, and isoflurane in a patient taking an antipsychotic drug can also cause a profound hypotensive reaction; therefore, this

Table 5–1.
Drug Interactions With Antipsychotics (Neuroleptics)

Combination	Interaction	Mechanism/ Comment	Clinical Significance
Angiotensin converting enzyme (ACE) ilnhibitors (captopril, enalopril) with CPZ	Pharmacologic effects of ACE inhibitors may be enhanced (marked hypotension)	Additive or synergistic pharmacologic activity Interaction: rapid onset	Yes
Anesthetics (enflurane, isoflurane, halothane with PTZ	Hypotension	? Potentiation of vasodilation myocardial depression	Yes
Anorexiants (e.g., amphetamine,.dextroamphetamine, phenmetrazine with CPZ, thioridazine, haloperidol	Diminished pharmacologic effects of amphetamines and congeners	Mechanism unknown	Yes
	Amphetamines may exacerbate psychotic symptoms		Yes
Gel-type antacids with Al^{+} and Mg^{+}	Decreased PTZ effect	Impaired GI absorption Clinical significance: charcoal only? Case report: haloperidol + antacid may lead to similar interaction	?
Anticholinergics (e.g.,benztropine [Cogentin], procyclidine [Kemadrin] trihexyphenidyl [Artane]) with CPZ, thioridazine, perphenazine, haloperidol	Delayed onset of antipsychotic effect in acute oral dose May decrease antipsychotic blood levels ↑ Anticholinergic adverse effects/ toxicity when used with PTZ (adynamic ileus, heat stroke, etc.)	Anticholinergics probably antagonize PTZ by direct CNS cholinergic pathways Anticholinergics may reduce GI absorption of CPZ, etc. Anticholinergic-type antiparkinsonin drugs are effective treatment for extrapyramidal reactions (parkinsonism)	Yes

Anticoagulants (e.g., warfarin)-CPZ	PTZ may potentiate action of warfarin	↓ metabolism (enzyme competition?)	?
		Haloperidol has been reported to lower anticoagulant effect of phenindione through enzyme induction	
Antidepressants			
Tricyclic (TCA) (e.g., imipramine,nortriptyline, desipramine) with PTZ, haloperidol	↑ Plasma levels of both drugs. (may ↑ CNS depression, and anticholinergic effect)	Possibly competitive inhibition of metabolism	Yes
	↑ Clinical efficacy (psychotic depression) and toxicity	? Synergism at CNS receptor site	Yes
		Depot antipsychotic might have the same effect as oral preparations	
		Avoid combination in high doses; decrease TCA dose if adverse effects are noted	
Monoamine oxidase inhibitors–PTZ (see also Chapr 2; Table 1–2)	↑ Hypotension	α-Adrenergic blockade and direct vasodilation	?
Antidiabetics-PTZ	PTZ may ↑ blood glucose	PTZs affect carbohydrate metabolism?	?
–	Insulin may ↑ brain level of CPZ(?)	↑ Required dose of diabetic medication if needed	
Antihypertensives			
Guanethidine (Ismelin), clonidine (Catapres) with PTZ, haloperidol, thiothixene	↓ Antihypertensive effect	Various antipsychotics may inhibit amine (guanethidine) uptake into adrenergic neuron	Yes
		Avoid the combination if possible	
		Reserpine, bethanidine, and debrisoquine have the same interaction	

(Continued.)

Table 5–1 (cont.).

Combination	Interaction	Mechanism/ Comment	Clinical Significance
		Molindone may be acceptable for patients receiving guanethidine-like antihypertensives Enhanced antihypertensive effect of clonidine has been reported with CPZ and fluphenazine	
α-Methyldopa (Aldomet) with PTZ	Marked hypotension	PTZs block α-adrenergic activity and α-methyldopa potentiates hypotension by formation of false transmitters	Yes
α-Methyldopa with haloperidol	↑ Risk of neurotoxicity, e.g., delirium (?)	Mechanism ? (2 case reports)	?
Antiparkinsonian drugs			
Anticholinergic types (see Anticholinergics)			
Levodopa	↓ Levodopa antiparkinsonian effect May exacerbate psychosis	Antagonism at receptor site	Yes
Ascorbic acid–Fluphenazine	↓ Fluphenazine pharmacologic and therapeutic action	Ascorbic acid may interfere with GI absorption of fluphenazine or stimulate hepatic metabolism (?) Single case report	?

Barbiturates Phenobarbital with PTZ, haloperidol	↓ Plasma antipsychotic levels ↑ Sedation	↑ Antipsychotic metabolism (induction of microsomal enzymes)	?
Barbiturate anesthetics (e.g., methohexital [Brevital], thiopental [Pentothal]) with PTZ	↑ Frequency and severity of neuromuscular excitation and hypotension	Mechanism Avoid preanesthetic administration of promethazine (Phenergan) in patients who receive methohexital or thiopental anesthesia Use other PTZs with caution in combination with these barbiturate anesthetics	Yes
β-blockers (propranolol [Inderal]) with PTZ	↑ Plasma levels and effect of both drugs	CPZ may inhibit hepatic metabolism of propranolol Mechanism of how propranolol affects PTZ is unknown Case report documents coadministration of haloperidol and propranolol causing hypotension and cardiopulmonary arrest	?
Benzodiazepines	↑ CNS sedation Benzodiazepines are effective in treatment of antipsychotic-induced acute dystonia and akathisia	? Mechanism	? Yes

(Continued.)

Table 5–1 (cont.).

Combination	Interaction	Mechanism/ Comment	Clinical Significance
Bromocriptine (Parlodel)-thioridazine	↓ Bromocriptine effect Bromocriptine may exacerbate psychosis.	Antagonism at receptor sites Avoid this combination if possible	?
Carbamazepine (see Chap 2, Table 2–1)			
Cigarette smoking–CPZ	↓ Antipsychotic effect(?)	↑ CPZ metabolism	?
Corticosteroids; digoxin	May enhance absorption of corticosteroids and digoxin	Various antipsychotics reduce . gut motility Space out dosage of 2 drugs as far as possible	
Diazoxide (Proglycem, Hyperstrat IV)-CPZ	May increase hyperglycemic effect of diazoxide	? Mechanism Single case report Use a PTZ with a lower potential for producing hyperglycemia in place of CPZ	?
Disulfiram (Antabuse) with PTZ, perphenazine (oral)	May ↓ perphenazine plasma levels	? Mechanism Single case report	?
Epinephrine, norepinephrine (Adrenalin, Levophed) with CPZ	CPZ decreases pressor effect of norepinephrine CPZ antagonizes peripheral vasoconstrictive effect of epinephrine	α-Adrenergic blockade and β-adrenergic stimulation	Yes

Ethanol (alcohol, other CNS depressants) with PTZ	Enhanced CNS depression Dystonic reactions may be precipitated by alcohol	Additive sedation? Alcohol may lower threshold of resistance to neurotoxic side effects of PTZ, or alter absorption of antipsychotic and increase plasma levels which leads to the unwanted effects Haloperidol may increase blood alcohol level, but not CPZ	Yes
Fluoxetine-haloperidol (see Chap 1)			
Griseofulvin, benzoquine, rifampin, phenylbutazone, dichloralphenazone	May ↓ effect of antipsychotic	↑ Antipsychotic metabolism	?
Hydantoins Phenytoin (Dilantin)-PTZ			
	May decrease phenytoin levels or increase phenytoin levels and toxicity	↓ Phenytoin levels by inducing liver enzyme?	?
Phenytoin-haloperidol	May ↓ serum concentration of haloperidol	↑ Metabolism of haloperidol (?)	?
Hydroxyzine (Atarax) with PTZ, CPZ, trifluoperazine	May ↓ antipsychotic effect of PTZ	? Mechanism	?
Lithium–PTZ, haloperidol (see Chap 2; Table 2–2)			

(Continued.)

Table 5–1 (cont.).

Combination	Interaction	Mechanism/ Comment	Clinical Significance
Metrizamide (Amipaque)-PTZ	May increase the possibility of seizure	Lowering of seizure threshold by combination has been proposed	
		Discontinue PTZ therapy at least 48 hr in advance of metrizamide use	Yes
		If seizure occurs, phenobarbitasl may be antiseizure drug of choice	
Narcotics, (e.g., meperidine [Demerol] with PTZ	Increased sedation	Additive CNS depressant and and cardiovascular effects	Yes
	Analgesia, hypotension, respiratory depression augmented	Benefit-to-risk ratio does not support administering this combination	
	Anticholinergic effects augmented by meperidine		
Oral contraceptives, chloramphenicol	May ↑ effect of neuroleptic drug	↓ Metabolism	?
Estrogen-containing contraceptives		May ↑ antipsychotic-induced prolactin stimulation	
Acetaminophen			
Orphenadrine-PTZ	↑ Hypoglycemic effect	Additive effect ?	?

Polypeptide antibiotics (polymyxin B [Aerosporin], bacitracin) with PTZ	May ↑ risk of respiratory paralysis	? Mechanism Case reports Animal study suggests possibility that these drugs could produce the same effect when administered alone	?
Quinidine-PTZ (e.g., thioridazine)	Cardiac arrhythmias, myocardial depression	Additive myocardial and electrophysiologic effects	?
Succinylcholine (Anectine)-PTZ	Prolonged neuromuscular blockade	? PTZ decreases levels of cholinesterase	?
Sympathomimetics (e.g., phenylpropanolamine [Propagest] with thioridazine)	May enhance ability of PTZ to produce arrhythmias	? Mechanism With sympathomimetics having both α and β-adrenergic activity, e.g., epinephrine, antipsychotic blockade of α-receptor may lead to unopposed β-receptor predominance, resulting in severe hypotension Levarterenol or phenylephrine may be safer	?
Valproic acid (Depakene) with PTZ, CPZ	↑ Plasma levels of valproic acid	CPZ may inhibit valproic acid metabolism Combination may have synergistic adverse effects (e.g., hepatic dysfunction) Haloperidol appears to be a better drug to use with valproic acid	?

drug combination should be avoided. The combination of narcotic and antipsychotic results in enhanced respiratory depression, hypotension, sedation, and analgesia. With meperidine, increased anticholinergic effects may occur. Numerous drugs exert a pronounced anticholinergic effect. For instance, most antiparkinsonian agents exert their action as a result of cholinergic blockade. Tricyclic and heterocyclic antidepressants produce marked anticholinergic action. Among antipsychotic agents, CPZ, thioridazine, and mesoridazine are most likely to produce significant cholinergic blockade. Since patients receiving antipsychotic drugs frequently are also receiving antiparkinsonian medication, and not unusually, TCAs as well, there is a strong likelihood of the patient experiencing excessive cholinergic blockade (blurred vision, dry mouth, tachycardia, constipation, urinary retention, stuttering speech, and impairment of memory and concentration) as a result of these combined regimens.

Many over-the-counter cold remedies, tranquilizers, and sleeping medications contain potent anticholinergic agents and antihistamines. Clinicians should be aware that coadministration of a variety of psychotropic drugs and over-the-counter medications may heighten the risk of an anticholinergic delirium or of peripheral manifestations of cholinergic blockade. CPZ has some ability to block nerve reuptake mechanisms and may therefore antagonize the antihypertensive effects of clonidine, guanethidine, and related drugs. Other significant interactions involving antipsychotic drugs and antihypertensives have been reported. Haloperidol combined with methyldopa may cause transient dementia. Some PTZs, most notably CPZ and thioridazine, can cause additive myocardial depression and dysrhythmias with quinidine, presumably due to the fact that both drugs exert similar electrophysiologic effects on the myocardium. Haloperidol has been used in a number of studies in rather high dosage in patients following acute myocardial infarction or open heart surgery. However, interactions with cardiac drugs and significant ECG effects have not been reported. Concomitant administration with antacids, activated charcoal, or cholestyramine may decrease the GI absorption and pharmacologic effects of PTZ. Many fruit juices and other beverages when mixed with liquid PTZ can result in the formation of an insoluble precipitate whose GI absorption appears to be impaired. Liquid preparations of haloperidol are compatible with beverages, and do not form insoluble precipitates with them. Although no longer marketed, iproniazid may decrease antipsychotic effects and its combination with an antipsychotic drug can produce hepatic toxicity and encephalopathy. PTZs should not be administered along with angiotensin converting enzyme (ACE) inhibitors, such as captopril or enalapril. Profound, symptomatic hypotension was reported in a patient concomitantly receiving CPZ and captopril.

PTZs may lower the seizure threshold and produce the need for adjustment of anticonvulsant doses in patients with seizure disorders. Despite the fact that there is no consistent evidence that PTZs are teratogenic, they may affect the developing nervous system and in animals they have been shown to have prolonged behavioral teratogenic effects.

Withdrawal Reactions. Tolerance develops to many of the untoward effects of the PTZs. Thus, when the drug is discontinued, rebound effects can occur. These effects can include insomnia, nightmares, anxiety, and cholinergic rebound effects, such as increased salivation, diarrhea, GI cramping, and vomiting. Furthermore, as discussed previously, withdrawal of the PTZ may produce a withdrawal dyskinesia that resembles tardive dyskinesia but which resolves with time.

Dosage and Administration

Choice of Agent. The choice of a specific agent is usually determined by the patients' past response, along with an understanding of the pharmacokinetics and side effects associated with each agent. In general, the high-potency phenothiazines tend to be less sedating than the low-potency agents and are associated with more extrapyramidal symptoms. Low-potency neuroleptics have strong anticholinergic and α-adrenergic blocking effects that tend to preclude their use in certain patient populations, e.g., the elderly.

Dosage. Dosage should be titrated to the individual's need and tolerance. The lowest effective dose should be used. After control of symptoms, dosage should be slowly titrated down to the minimally effective dose. Early in the treatment course, dividing doses into two to three doses can reduce the incidence of side effects. Due to the long half-lives of most PTZs and their typically slow onset of action, the clinician should continue any individual medication for a period of weeks before determining whether or not a trial is adequate.

As the psychotic symptoms resolve, consideration must be given to maintenance treatment. Again, the lowest effective dose should be used. Based on the evidence available, it appears that most patients with chronic schizophrenia need long-term maintenance treatment to prevent relapses. The patient should be reevaluated periodically during long-term treatment, however, both for evaluation of the continued need for the drug and for the development of side effects.

In the next section, the individual antipsychotic agents are listed in alphabetical order with specific comments provided on the pharmacology, uses, cautions, dosage, administration, and preparations available of each agent.

ACETOPHENAZINE MALEATE

Chemical Class: Piperazine Phenothiazine

Pharmacology

Acetophenazine has weak anticholinergic effects, moderate to severe extrapyramidal effects, and is moderately sedating. Its pharmacologic effects are otherwise similar to those of CPZ.

Pharmacokinetics

Acetophenazine is readily absorbed from the GI tract and is highly bound to plasma proteins. It undergoes hepatic metabolism followed by renal and hepatic excretion.

Uses

Acetophenazine is used in the treatment of psychosis and provides symptomatic relief in most patients. Those who do not respond to acetophenazine should be tried on an alternative neuroleptic.

Cautions

The general precautions regarding the use of phenothiazines should be observed for acetophenazine. (See the General Statement regarding cautions in the use of PTZs.)

Dosage and Administration

Dosage. Acetophenazine 20 mg is the therapeutic equivalent of 2 mg of haloperidol. As with all neuroleptics, the dosage should be titrated to the individual's need and tolerance. After treatment of acute symptomatology, the dosage should be titrated to the lowest clinically effective amount. When treating the elderly or debilitated, the dosage should be gradually increased as tolerated. Geriatric patients may respond to a lower dose than that used for young, healthy adults. In addition, outpatients generally receive lower doses than acutely ill inpatients.

The usual adult dosage is 20 mg 3 times a day. Acetophenazine is somewhat sedating, and for that reason the last dose may be administered at bedtime for those patients who have difficulty sleeping. For severely ill patients, dosage may range from 80 to 120 mg/day in divided doses. Inpatient dosages for severely ill patients range as high as 600 mg/day.

Administration. Acetophenazine maleate is administered orally.

Preparations

Acetophenazine maleate (*Tindal*)
  Oral tablets
    20 mg

CHLORPROMAZINE HYDROCHLORIDE

Chemical Class: Aliphatic Phenothiazine

Pharmacology

CPZ has mild to moderate extrapyramidal effects and strong sedative and anticholinergic effects. It is a powerful antiemetic and a strong adrenergic blocking agent. It has weak antihistaminic and antiserotonergic activity.

Pharmacokinetics

Absorption. CPZ is rapidly absorbed from parenteral injection sites and from the GI tract. However, following absorption it undergoes considerable metabolism in the GI mucosa and significant first-pass metabolism in the liver. There is considerable variation in plasma concentrations produced in different individuals receiving the same dose. This may represent genetic differences in the rate of first-pass metabolism.

Distribution. CPZ is 95% bound to plasma proteins. CPZ and its metabolites cross the placenta and are found in human breast milk.

Elimination. CPZ undergoes extensive metabolism with approximately 10 to 12 active metabolites. Metabolism includes hydroxylation and demethylation. Two principle groups of metabolites occur: the first is an unconjugated fraction representing about 20% of CPZ and its metabolites; the remaining portion is the conjugated fraction.

Uses

CPZ is used in the treatment of schizophrenia, the manic phase of bipolar disorder, and the treatment of nausea and vomiting.

Cautions

CPZ shares the toxicity of other neuroleptics. (See the General Statement on PTZs.) Some preparations of CPZ contain sulfites that may cause an allergic reaction including anaphylaxis and severe asthmatic episodes in certain individuals. Sulfite sensitivity is more common in asthmatic than nonasthmatic individuals.

Dosage and Administration

Dosage. CPZ 100 mg is the therapeutic equivalent of 2 mg of haloperidol. Dosage must be titrated to the individual's need and tolerance. Lower initial dosages and more gradual augmentation in dosage should be used in geriatric or medically ill patients since the risk of most side effects is dose-related. Geriatric patients are particularly sensitive to anticholinergic side effects and to α-adrenergic blockade. The latter may cause orthostatic hypotension with the secondary risk of falling and hip fracture. There should be regular assessment of clinical indications along with evaluation of the development of possible side effects in patients receiving long-term therapy. The usual initial dosage in nonhospitalized patients is 25 mg three times a day which is gradually increased until symptoms are controlled. While some symptomatic relief may occur during the first week of treatment, many patients will require 1 week or more until optimum control is achieved.

Many patients will be adequately treated with approximately 200 mg/day on an outpatient basis. However, oral dosages of up to 800 mg/day may be required in some severe cases. Many inpatients will be maintained on 500 mg/day. Generally, there is little additional therapeutic gain achieved when dosages greater than 1 g/day are given for prolonged periods The usual initial dose for hospitalized patients is 25 mg three times a day, although in more severe cases of agitation 25- to 50-mg dosages may be given as frequently as every hour intramuscularly (IM). IM injections may produce significant hypotension and local irritation. If IM administration is required, many practitioners prefer to use high-potency neuroleptics.

In children, the initial dose for treatment of psychiatric disorders is usually 0.55 mg/kg every 4 to 6 hours as needed. This is true for both oral and IM preparations. For rectal administration the usual administration in children is 1.1 mg/kg every 6 to 8 hours as needed. The maximum IM dosage of CPZ in children less than 5 years of age is 40 mg/day; in children from 5 to 12 years of age dosage should not exceed 75 mg/day.

For the treatment of nausea or vomiting the usual oral administration is 10 to 25 mg every 4 to 6 hours; the usual rectal dose is 100 mg every 6 to 8 hours or 25 mg IM every 3 to 4 hours as needed. For intractable hiccups the usual dose is 25 to 50 mg 3 to 4 times a day; IM administration may be used in the same dosages if symptoms persist for 2 to 3 days.

Administration. Chlorpromazine hydrochloride may be administered orally or by IM or intravenous (IV) injection. IV injection is used during surgery to control nausea and vomiting, and IV infusion is used in the treatment of intractable hiccups. Owing to the possibility of hypotension, patients receiving parenteral therapy should remain recumbent for at least 30 minutes after drug administration. CPZ (as the base) is administered rectally.

Preparation

Chlorpromazine hydrochloride
- Rectal suppositories (*Thorazine*)
  - 25 mg, 100 mg
- Capsules, extended-release (*Thorazine, Spansule*)
  - 30 mg, 75 mg, 100 mg, 200 mg, 300 mg
- Solution (*Thorazine Syrup*)
  - 10 mg/5 mL
- Solution, concentrate (*Intensol, Thorazine Concentrate*)
  - 30 mg/mL, 100 mg/mL
- Tablets (*Thorazine*)
  - 10 mg, 25 mg, 50 mg, 100 mg, 200 mg
- Parenteral injection (*Ormazine, Promaz, Thorazine*)
  - 25 mg/mL

The duration of action of the chlorpromazine hydrochloride tablet is approximately 4 to 6 hours. For the extended-release formulation the duration of action is 10 to 12 hours.

CHLORPROTHIXENE, CHLORPROTHIXENE HYDROCHLORIDE, CHLORPROTHIXENE LACTATE

Chemical Class: Thioxanthene

Pharmacology

Chlorprothixene has mild to moderate extrapyramidal effects, and strong antiemetic, anticholinergic, sedative, and hypothermic activities. It is a potent inhibitor of postural reflexes and motor coordination.

Pharmacokinetics

Chlorprothixene is partly absorbed from the GI tract after oral or IM administration. The drug is principally metabolized in the liver to chlorprothixene sulfoxide. Chlorprothixene and its metabolites are excreted in both urine and feces.

Uses

Chlorprothixene is used in the treatment of psychotic disorders.

Cautions

Chlorprothixene shares the potential for toxic reactions of PTZs. (See the General Statement on PTZs for details.)

Taractan tablets contain tartrazine (FD&C yellow no. 5). This may cause allergic reactions in certain individuals. Although the incidence of sensitivity to tartrazine is low, it most commonly occurs in patients who are sensitive to aspirin. The safety and efficacy of chlorprothixene have not been established in children younger than 12 years of age.

Dosage and Administration

Dosage. Chlorprothixene 100 mg is the therapeutic equivalent of 2 mg of haloperidol. Dosage should be titrated to the individual's need and tolerance. In addition, since some toxic side effects are related to prolonged use, patients receiving chronic chlorprothixene administration should be periodically reevaluated for the development of toxic side effects and to assess continued indication for treatment. The usual initial dose in adults is 25 to 50 mg three or four times daily, administered orally. The maximum oral dose of chlorprothixene rarely exceeds 600 mg/day. The usual initial oral dosage in children older than 12 years of age is 10 to 25 mg three or four times a day. In cases of acute agitation symptomatic management may be obtained using an initial IM dose of 25 to 50 mg repeated up to 3 or 4 times daily if necessary. Geriatric patients are particularly sensitive to anticholinergic side effects and to α-adrenergic blockade. The latter may cause orthostatic hypotension with the secondary risk of falling and hip fracture. After adequate behavioral control has been obtained using parenteral administration, the patient should be converted to oral agents as soon as possible.

Administration. Chlorprothixene and chlorprothixene hydrochloride are both administered orally. Chlorprothixene hydrochloride and lactate are administered as oral suspensions, and chlorprothixene hydrochloride is also administered by IM injection. The patient should be in a recumbent position for IM administration and be closely supervised for the development of orthostatic hypotension.

Preparations

Chlorprothixene (*Taractan*)
  Oral tablets
    10 mg, 25 mg, 50 mg, 100 mg
Chlorprothixene hydrochloride (*Taractan*)
  Parenteral injection
    12.5 mg/mL
Chlorprothixene hydrochloride and lactate (*Taractan concentrate*)
Oral suspension
    100 mg/5 mL

CLOZAPINE

Clozapine has unique properties compared with the other antipsychotics. It is not a neuroleptic; it does not appear to produce extrapyramidal symptoms or other antidopaminergic side effects. It does, however, have α-adrenergic blocking effects, anticholinergic effects, and sedative properties. It appears to be effective in the treatment of the negative symptoms of schizophrenia, i.e., apathy, social withdrawal, and flattened affect; this effect is unlike all other neuroleptics. Clozapine may be more effective than other drugs used for the treatment of psychosis; furthermore, it is associated with adverse effects that are quite different from those of the neuroleptics.

Pharmacology

While clozapine binds to both dopamine-1 (D_1) and -2 (D_2) receptors, the profile of dopamine binding and its effect on dopamine-mediated behaviors differs greatly from that of the typical antipsychotic drug. Clozapine is preferentially more active at limbic than at striatal dopamine receptors. Clozapine binds strongly to serotonin-2, α_1-adrenergic, muscarinic, and histamine $(H)_1$ receptors. D_1 and D_2 are blocked by clozapine to a lesser degree.

Pharmacokinetics

Peak serum levels occur approximately 1.5 to 2.5 hours after oral administration of clozapine. Food does not affect the bioavailability of clozapine. The drug is 95% bound to serum proteins. Interactions with other protein-bound drugs are unknown. The drug is metabolized prior to excretion; it is excreted in both urine and feces. The desmethyl metabolite has some pharmacologic activity. The mean elimination half-life of clozapine is 10 to 12 hours, with the elimination half-life increasing after multiple doses have been administered.

Uses

Clozapine is indicated in the treatment of schizophrenic patients who manifest severe symptomatology and who have had an inadequate response to traditional antipsychotic medications. Clozapine should only be used in those patients in whom there has been an inadequate response to appropriate courses of traditional antipsychotic drugs or where the patient has been unable to receive an adequate course because of inability to tolerate the adverse effects of these drugs. Clozapine has been shown to be superior to both haloperidol and CPZ in the treatment of drug-resistant, chronic schizophrenic patients with severe illness.

Contraindications

Clozapine should not be used in patients with severe granulocytopenia, a history of clozapine-induced agranulocytosis, or in patients with myeloproliferative disorders. Likewise, clozapine should not be concurrently administered to patients who are receiving agents which suppress bone marrow function.

Warnings. Because of the risk of seizures and agranulocytosis associated with the use of clozapine, this drug should only be provided to those patients who have failed to respond to adequate courses of standard antipsychotic drugs or who have been unable to tolerate a standard course because of intolerable side effects. The manufacturer strongly recommends that patients be given at least two trials of different standard antipsychotic drugs at adequate dosage durations prior to initiating treatment with clozapine. Patients are required to have a baseline WBC and differential count before the initiation of clozapine treatment. In addition, a WBC count must be obtained every week throughout treatment and every 4 weeks after the discontinuation of clozapine. Without these tests, the manufacturer will not continue to dispense the medication. This is because the incidence of agranulocytosis at 1 year is approximately 2%. The risk is highest between the 6th and 18th weeks of treatment. Therefore, blood tests may not actually be needed at this frequency after the 18th week.

Agranulocytosis is defined as a granulocyte count (polymorphonuclear and bandforms) of less than 500/mm^3. Agranulocytosis may be fatal if not recognized early and treated promptly. Treatment with clozapine should not be initiated if the WBC count is less than 3,500/mm^3, or if the patient has a history of a myeloproliferative disorder, a history of previous clozapine-induced agranulocytosis, or granulocytopenia. Patients should be cautioned to report promptly the development of fever, sore throat, weakness, lethargy, or other signs of infection. After initiation of clozapine, if the total WBC count falls below 3,000/mm^3, or if the granulocyte count falls below 1,500/mm^3, clozapine therapy should be discontinued. At that point, patients should be monitored for the development of symptoms consistent with an infection. If no infection develops, and the WBC total count returns to levels above 3,000/mm^3, and the granulocyte count returns to levels above 1,500/mm^3, then clozapine therapy may be resumed.

Twice-weekly WBC counts should be continued until total WBC counts return to above 3,500/mm^3. For those patients in whom the total WBC count drops to below 2,000/mm^3 or the granulocyte count falls to below 1,000/mm^3, a bone marrow aspiration should be considered to ascertain the granulopoietic status. Protective isolation may be necessary if granulopoiesis is insufficient. If, at that time, evidence suggestive of an infection develops, the patient should receive appropriate cultures followed by appropriate antibiotic treatment. In patients whose total WBC count has fallen below 2,000/mm^3 or whose granulocyte count has fallen below 1,000/mm^3 during a course of therapy, they should not be subsequently rechallenged with clozapine.

Seizures have been reported to occur with a cumulative 1-year incidence of approximately 4% in patients taking clozapine. Seizures are more likely to occur with higher dosages of clozapine. Care should be exercised in administering clozapine to patients with a history of seizure disorder or with factors predisposing to seizures. Patients should be cautioned about performing hazardous activities, such as operating large machinery or swimming, where sudden loss of consciousness could pose a serious risk to others or themselves.

Neuroendocrine effects of clozapine produce little or no prolactin elevation.

Clozapine increases delta and theta activity and slows dominant alpha frequencies on the EEG. There is enhanced synchronization and sharp-wave activity; spike and wave complexes may also occur.

Cardiovascular Effects. Clozapine has been associated with orthostatic hypotension which is more common during initial drug administration or after rapid dose increase. Some 25% of patients may develop tachycardia.

Neuroleptic malignant syndrome. No cases of NMS have been attributed to clozapine therapy alone. However, there have been cases of patients taking clozapine and other CNS-active agents who have developed NMS. (See the General Statement regarding PTZs for a description of NMS.)

Tardive Dyskinesia. For a description of tardive dyskinesia, see the General Statement regarding neuroleptics. There has been only one case of tardive dyskinesia developing during clozapine use. However, it cannot yet be concluded with certainty that clozapine is incapable of inducing this syndrome. Based on its weak dopamine-blocking effect and the virtual absence of acute extrapyramidal symptoms, there is reason to believe that clozapine may not cause tardive dyskinesia.

Cautions

General. Clozapine should be used for the briefest possible time to minimize the risk of development of agranulocytosis or seizures. For this reason, in patients who fail to show an acceptable level of clinical response, the drug trial should be kept brief, though some recent research suggests that some patients respond to clozapine only after several months and up to 1 year. Furthermore, in those patients who respond to clozapine, there should be an ongoing assessment of the need for continuing treatment. Clozapine should not be administered concurrently with other agents known to suppress bone marrow function. The mechanism of clozapine-induced agranulocytosis is unknown. Until this is elucidated, the possibility that such agents may interact in a synergistic manner to increase the risk or severity of bone marrow suppression should be considered.

Fever. Patients may experience transient fever greater than 38°C (100.4°F). This most commonly occurs during the first 3 weeks of treatment and is usually benign and self-limiting. However, when it occurs, patients should be evaluated for the possibility that there may be an increase or decrease in the WBC count, an underlying infectious process, or the development of NMS.

Anticholinergic Toxicity. Clozapine has strong anticholinergic effects. Patients should be assessed for the development of anticholinergic toxicity. Furthermore, the drug should be used with caution in those patients having conditions making them vulnerable to anticholinergic effects such as prostatic hypertrophy or narrow-angle glaucoma.

Interference With Cognitive and Motor Performance. During the first few days after initiation of clozapine therapy, many patients may experience sedation. This may be severe enough to impair mental or physical abilities, or both. During this period of time, and subsequently, patients should be cautioned about engaging in hazardous activities which require continued alertness.

Use in Patients With Concomitant Illness. There is limited experience in the administration of clozapine to patients with preexisting systemic diseases. For this reason, it is prudent to exercise caution in the administration of clozapine to a patient with hepatic, cardiac, or renal disease.

Drug Interactions. Clozapine may potentiate the anticholinergic effects of other atropine-like agents. Clozapine may also potentiate the hypotensive effects of antihypertensive drugs. Epinephrine should be avoided in the treatment of drug-induced hypotension because of a possible reverse epinephrine effect.

Distribution. Clozapine may be distributed in human breast milk and potentially have an effect on the infant.

Pediatric Use. The safety and efficacy of clozapine in children younger than 16 years of age have not been established.

Toxicity

Associated With Discontinuation of Treatment. Reactions that are associated with the discontinuation of clozapine have included drowsiness, sedation, seizures, dizziness or syncope, tachycardia, hypotension, ECG changes, nausea and vomiting, leukopenia, granulocytopenia, agranulocytosis, and fever. Each of these events accounted for less than 1.7% of all drug discontinuations attributed to adverse clinical events.

Commonly Observed. Adverse side effects associated with the use of clozapine that occurred with an incidence greater than 5% during preclinical trials of clozapine included drowsiness or sedation, dizziness or vertigo, headache and tremor, salivation, sweating, dry mouth, visual disturbances, tachycardia, hypotension, syncope, constipation, nausea, and fever. Drowsiness or sedation diminishes with continued drug administration. Salivation may be profuse and more common during sleep. It appears to be dose-responsive, diminishing with reduction in drug dosage; it may also respond to low doses of anticholinergic medication.

Overdosage. Fatal overdoses have been reported with doses greater than 2,500 mg. However, there have been reports of patients recovering from overdoses in excess of 4 g. Common manifestations of clozapine overdose include altered states of consciousness, which may include drowsiness progressing to delirium and subsequently coma. There may be tachycardia, hypotension, respiratory depression, and hypersalivation. Seizures have occurred in some cases.

Management of Overdose. After the establishment of an adequate airway, attempts should be made to remove as much of the drug as possible. This is best accomplished with lavage. Also, activated charcoal with sorbitol may be highly effective. Careful monitoring of vital signs and supportive measures should be undertaken. Epinephrine and its derivatives should be avoided as treatment for hypotension because of the possibility of a reverse epinephrine effect.

Dosage and Administration

Initial Treatment. The usual initial dose is 25 mg once or twice a day. Dosage may be increased by 25 or 50 mg/day as tolerated to achieve a dosage of 300 to 450 mg/day by the end of 2 weeks. After that dose range has been achieved, subsequent dose increments should be made no more often than once or twice weekly. Increases in dosage should not exceed 100 mg at a time. Hypotension, seizure, and sedation may be minimized by using a divided dose schedule and careful dose titration. (See also under How Supplied below.)

Therapeutic Dose Adjustment. During dose titration, daily dosing should continue on a divided basis. Many patients will respond adequately to doses between 300 and 600 mg/day. However, for some patients it may be necessary to increase the dose to between 600 and 900 mg/day. In general, dosage should not exceed 900 mg/day. In addition, sufficient time should be given for the patient to respond to a particular dose level before further increases are attempted. In order to minimize the risk of agranulocytosis and seizure, patients who fail to show an acceptable level of response should not be maintained on extended treatment.

Maintenance Treatment. Patients who respond to clozapine should be maintained on the lowest clinically effective dose needed to maintain remission. They should be periodically reassessed for continued indication for drug treatment and for the development of toxic side effects.

Discontinuation of Treatment. A gradual reduction in dose is recommended rather than abrupt discontinuation of clozapine. This gradual reduction should occur over a period of 1 to 2 weeks. If there is a medical condition which requires abrupt discontinuation, such as leukopenia, the patient should be carefully observed for the development of psychotic symptomatology.

How Supplied. Clozapine is available as round tablets, 25 and 100 mg; in a ten-tablet (25-mg) pack, *Sandopak*; and in a 100-mg 10-tablet *Sandopak*. Clozapine is also available in total daily dose packages. Each contains 1 week's medication: 150 mg/day, containing two 25-mg and one 100-mg tablets; and 200 mg/day, 250 mg/day, 300 mg/day, 400 mg/day, 500 mg/day, and 600 mg/day packages. The proprietary name for clozapine is *Clozaril*.

DROPERIDOL

Chemical Class: Butyrophenone

Pharmacology

The pharmacologic actions of droperidol are similar to those of haloperidol. Droperidol has strong sedative and antiemetic effects, a moderate tendency to produce extrapyramidal reactions, and weak anticholinergic and antiadrenergic effects.

Pharmacokinetics

Absorption. The onset of action occurs approximately 3 to 10 minutes after IM or IV administration. The acute sedative effects usually last for less than 4 hours. However, effects may persist for up to 12 hours.

Elimination. Droperidol is metabolized in the liver to *p*-fluorophenylacetic acid which is then conjugated and excreted in urine and feces. Less than 10% of the unmetabolized drug is excreted.

Uses

Droperidol is used for the symptomatic management of acute psychotic disorders. It is not intended for long term administration. Droperidol is also commonly used as an adjunct to anesthesia and as an antiemetic.

Cautions

The cautions which apply to droperidol are similar to those of haloperidol.

Cardiovascular Effects. Transient, mild hypotension is the most frequent adverse effect associated with droperidol. Occasionally tachycardia may occur.

CNS Effects. Extrapyramidal reactions, most commonly consisting of dystonia and akathisia, may occur. Less frequent reactions include chills and shivering.

Precautions and Contraindications. The toxic potential of droperidol is similar to that of PTZs. (See the General Statement on PTZs for details.) Droperidol should be used with caution in patients with impaired renal or hepatic function.

Acute Toxicity. In general, the manifestations of overdosage are extensions of the general pharmacologic actions of droperidol. Treatment is supportive and symptomatic. In particular, hypotension and hypoventilation should be managed. Vital signs should be monitored regularly and body temperature maintained. In addition, adequate fluids should be administered to minimize hypotension.

Dosage and Administration

Dosage. Dosage should be titrated to the individual's need and tolerance. The usual IM dose is 2.5 to 10 mg. IV injection should not exceed 100 mg twice daily.

Administration. Droperidol is administered either IM or IV. IV administration is usually reserved for acute psychosis where large amounts of medication need to be quickly administered. IM administration is used on those occasions when IV administration is not possible or when doses smaller than 10 mg are indicated.

Preparations

Droperidol (*Inapsine*)
  Parenteral injection
    2.5 mg/mL

FLUPHENAZINE DECANOATE, FLUPHENAZINE ENANTHATE, FLUPHENAZINE HYDROCHLORIDE

Chemical Class: Piperazine Phenothiazine

Pharmacology

Fluphenazine is more potent than CPZ and has weak anticholinergic, sedative, and antiemetic effects. It has prominent extrapyramidal effects. Its general pharmacologic actions are similar to those of CPZ.

Pharmacokinetics

Fluphenazine hydrochloride is rapidly absorbed from both parenteral injection sites and the GI tract. The duration of action is approximately 6 to 8 hours. Fluphenazine decanoate or fluphenazine enanthate have an onset of action within 24 to 72 hours and a duration of action from 1 to 6 weeks with an average of 2 weeks. The decanoate ester may last slightly longer than the enanthate ester. Rate of release of the drug is slowed both by esterification and by administration of these esters in a sesame oil vehicle.

Uses

Fluphenazine is used to manage psychotic disorders. The advantage of the long-acting decanoate and enanthate esters is with the maintenance treatment of patients with chronic schizophrenia who do not reliably take oral antipsychotic agents. Should complications arise, there is no ability to terminate the drug effect of these long-acting preparations. The long-acting form should not be used for acute symptomatic control. Some individuals appear to have a preferential response to one antipsychotic as opposed to another; those individuals who do not respond to fluphenazine should be tried on alternative therapeutic agents.

Cautions

See the General Statement on toxicity with PTZs.

Fluphenazine has a tendency to produce extrapyramidal reactions. These are more likely to occur with long-acting forms of the drug. They usually occur after the first 2 to 3 days post administration and may last for approximately 5 days.

Prolixin tablets, 2.5 mg, 5 mg, and 10 mg, contain tartrazine dye (FD&C yellow no. 5); this may cause allergic reactions or bronchial asthma in susceptible individuals. Tartrazine sensitivity most commonly occurs in patients who are sensitive to aspirin. The use of depot preparations of fluphenazine has not been established to be safe or efficacious in children under the age of 12 years.

Dosage and Administration

Dosage. Fluphenazine is approximately equipotent to haloperidol. Dosage must be titrated to the individual's need and tolerance because adverse consequences are more likely to occur with long-term administration of the drug. Patients on chronic fluphenazine treatment should be periodically reevaluated for the development of toxic side effects and for indication for continued drug treatment. The usual dosage for psychotic adults is 2.5 to 10 mg daily. In most cases optimum therapeutic effect occurs with dosages at or under 20 mg/day. Dosages up to 40 mg/day may be required for brief periods of time in severely disturbed patients. However, caution should be used in exceeding 20 mg/day of fluphenazine.

After control of acute symptoms, dosage should be titrated to the lowest possible effective dose. In most cases the usual IM dose of fluphenazine hydrochloride is approximately one-third to one-half the oral dose. The initial total IM dosage of fluphenazine may range from 2.5 to 10 mg/day given in divided doses every 6 to 8 hours. Dosage is then titrated as indicated until symptoms are controlled. In general, IM dosages which exceed 10 mg/day should be used with caution. As soon as possible, oral therapy should replace parenteral administration.

In patients who have not received a trial with PTZs, it is recommended that they first receive a trial of fluphenazine hydrochloride prior to the administration of fluphenazine decanoate or fluphenazine enanthate. This is done to determine the patient's approximate dosage and document and determine susceptibility to any adverse effects. There is no precise formula for converting fluphenazine hydrochloride to either fluphenazine decanoate or fluphenazine enanthate. However, many believe that 20 mg/day of fluphenazine hydrochloride is approximately equivalent to 25 mg of fluphenazine decanoate every 2 weeks. This conversion represents a ratio of 12.5 mg of fluphenazine decanoate every 2 weeks for every 10 mg of fluphenazine hydrochloride daily. In most cases, the usual IM or subcutaneous dose of fluphenazine decanoate is 12.5 to 25 mg every 2 weeks. The usual initial IM or subcutaneous dosage of fluphenazine enanthate is 25 mg every 2 weeks. Subsequently, dosage must be titrated to the individual's need and response.

Administration. Fluphenazine hydrochloride is administered orally or by IM injection. Fluphenazine enanthate and fluphenazine decanoate are administered by IM or subcutaneous injection. The fluphenazine hydrochloride oral concentrate solution must be diluted prior to administration.

Preparations

Fluphenazine decanoate (*Prolixin Decanoate*)
- Parenteral injection
  - 25 mg/mL

Fluphenazine enanthate
- Parenteral injection (*Prolixin Enanthate*)
  - 25 mg/mL
- Oral elixir (*Prolixin*)
  - 2.5 mg/5 mL
- Solution, concentrate (*Permitil, Prolixin*)
  - 5 mg/mL

Tablets

1 mg (Prolixin), 2.5 mg, 5.0 mg, 10 mg (Permitil, Proxilin)

Fluphenazine hydrochloride (*Prolixin*)

Parenteral injection (for IM use only)

2.5 mg/mL

HALOPERIDOL, HALOPERIDOL LACTATE, HALOPERIDOL DECANOATE

Chemical Class: Butyrophenone

Pharmacology

Haloperidol appears to have strong antidopaminergic activity and has weak anticholinergic activity. It may cause extrapyramidal reactions, but it produces less hypotension, sedation, and hypothermia than CPZ. The pharmacologic effects of haloperidol are similar to those of the piperazine phenothiazines; however, the chemical structures of the butyrophenones and piperazines are unrelated.

Pharmacokinetics

Absorption. Haloperidol is well absorbed from the GI tract following oral administration. There is extensive first-pass liver metabolism with approximately 40% being metabolized. Maximum pharmacologic action occurs approximately 30 to 45 minutes after IM administration.

Haloperidol decanoate is esterified haloperidol. Esterification prolongs the duration of action by resulting in a slow and gradual release of the drug from fatty tissues. The ester is administered in sesame oil to further delay the rate of release. Peak plasma levels occur approximately 1 week after IM haloperidol decanoate administration. Steady-state concentrations in serum are reached in approximately 4 months following once-monthly IM injections.

Distribution. Approximately 92% of haloperidol is bound to plasma proteins. Haloperidol is also distributed into breast milk.

Elimination. Haloperidol is principally metabolized in the liver by oxidative N-dealkylation and by reduction. The reduced metabolite hydroxyhaloperidol may have pharmacologic activity. Haloperidol and its metabolites are excreted in urine and feces.

Haloperidol decanoate is slowly released from fatty tissue. Subsequently, hydrolysis occurs by plasma and tissue esterases to produce decanoic acid and haloperidol. From this point on, metabolism is similar to that of the orally administered drug. IM decanoate has an approximate half-life of 3 weeks.

Uses

Haloperidol is used for the control of psychotic disorders. Individual response to this particular neuroleptic may vary. Those individuals who fail to fully respond to one drug should be tried on alternative compounds. The long-acting decanoate form is used for those individuals who require long-term antipsychotic therapy, particularly patients with a history of poor compliance with oral medication. Long-acting forms should not be used for acute patient management. Most patients are usually stabilized first on oral haloperidol and then subsequently converted to IM haloperidol decanoate. This minimizes the possibility of an unexpected adverse reaction that could not readily be reversed with decanoate therapy. Long-acting preparations may also be useful in patients with GI malabsorption. Haloperidol is also useful for the control of tics and Gilles de la Tourette's syndrome in both children and adults.

Cautions

The toxic potential of haloperidol is similar to that of other antipsychotic agents. (See the General Statement regarding PTZs for details.) Haloperidol may produce hypotension. For this reason, it should be used with caution in those patients with severe cardiovascular disorders. Haloperidol may lower the seizure threshold and should be used with caution in patients with a known seizure disorder. Patients should be cautioned that haloperidol may impair the ability to perform activities which require physical coordination or mental alertness. Haldol tablets, 1 mg, 5 mg, and 10 mg, contain tartrazine (FD&C yellow no. 5). This may produce an allergic reaction in some sensitive individuals. The incidence of tartrazine sensitivity is higher in patients who are sensitive to aspirin. The safety and efficacy of haloperidol decanoate has not been established in children. Likewise, the safety and efficacy of other preparations in children younger than 3 years of age have not been established.

Extrapyramidal Reactions. Extrapyramidal symptoms are frequent with haloperidol. These most commonly occur in the first few days of therapy. Akathisia, dystonic reactions, and a parkinsonian syndrome are common. The occurrence and severity of extrapyramidal reactions is usually dose-related and will therefore improve with reduction in the administered dose. In some cases anticholinergic or antiparkinsonian medication may be of help. Tardive dyskinesia may occur in patients who receive long-term administration of the drug. Transient withdrawal dyskinesia may occur with abrupt discontinuation of antipsychotic agents in patients who have received prolonged treatment. In some patients there may be galactorrhea and gynecomastia.

Toxicity

The manifestations of a haloperidol overdosage are extensions of its common adverse reactions. Most often this includes severe extrapyramidal reactions, hypotension, and sedation. Coma, hypotension, respiratory depression, and prolongation of the QT interval may occur. Treatment consists of symptomatic and supportive care. Anticholinergic antiparkinsonian agents may help control extrapyramidal reactions. If possible, the stomach should be emptied by gastric lavage. Activated charcoal should be administered after gastric emptying. Hypotension or excessive sedation should be appropriately treated. Epinephrine should not be used for hypotension.

Dosage and Administration

Dosage. Dosage should be titrated to the lowest effective clinical dose. Lower dosages may be used in children and in the geriatric population. The risk of adverse reactions increases with duration of drug use, and for this reason, patients on chronic drug treatment should receive periodic examinations to assess development of toxic side effects and continued indication for drug treatment. For management of Gilles de la Tourette's syndrome, moderate psychotic disorders in adults, or treatment in the geriatric population, the usual initial dosage is 0.5 to 2.0 mg 2 to 3 times a day. Dosage is subsequently titrated to the individual's need and tolerance.

The usual initial dosage for patients with severe symptomatology is 5 to 10 mg 2 to 3 times per day.

The usual IM dose is 5 to 10 mg for acute agitation. This may be repeated as needed as often as every hour. However, in most cases administration every 4 to 8 hours is adequate. Parenteral therapy should be replaced by oral therapy as soon as possible. For IM decanoate an initial adult dosage is 10 to 15 times the previous daily dose of oral haloperidol; this should not exceed 100 mg. Haloperidol decanoate is usually administered once every 4 weeks. However, dosage should be titrated to the individual's need and tolerance.

The usual initial oral dosage of haloperidol in children weighing between 15 and 40 kg and between 3 and 12 years of age is 0.5 mg/day given in 2 or 3 divided doses. Dosage may be increased by 0.5 mg depending on indications and tolerance. In the case of severe psychotic disorders in children in this age range, the initial dosage may be 0.05 to 0.15 mg/kg/day given in 2 or 3 divided doses. In Gilles de la Tourette's syndrome in children 3 to 12 years of age, the usual dosage is 0.05 to 0.075 mg/kg/day.

Administration. Haloperidol is administered orally. Haloperidol lactate is administered either orally or by IM injection. Haloperidol decanoate is administered by IM injection.

Preparations

Haloperidol
- Oral tablets
  - 0.5 mg, 1 mg, 2 mg, 5 mg,
  - 20 mg (*Haldol*), 10 mg (*Halperon*)
- Tablets, film-coated
  - 0.5 mg, 1 mg, 2 mg, 5 mg

Haloperidol decanoate
- Parenteral injection
  - 50 mg/mL

Haloperidol lactate
- Oral solution (*Haldol Concentrate, Haloperidol Intensol, Myperidol*)
  - 2 mg/mL
- Parenteral injection (*Haldol*)
  - 5 mg/mL

LOXAPINE HYDROCHLORIDE, LOXAPINE SUCCINATE

Chemical Class: Dibenzoxapine

Pharmacology

The pharmacologic actions of loxapine are similar to those of the PTZs. In patients with known seizure disorders, loxapine has induced generalized tonoclonic seizures in the usual therapeutic dose range. Antiemetic activity has not been systematically evaluated in humans. Loxapine has moderate to severe extrapyramidal effect, with moderate anticholinergic and antiadrenergic effect.

Pharmacokinetics

Absorption. Loxapine is almost entirely absorbed from the GI tract with peak plasma concentrations occurring approximately 2 hours after administration; with IM injection this is reduced to 1 hour. The drug is metabolized to 8-hydroxyloxapine which is an active metabolite, and 8-hydroxyamoxapine which has antidepressant activity, though probably not clinically significant at the low concentrations achieved with loxapine administration. Peak effects after oral administration occur in approximately 1.5 to 3.0 hours with the duration of effects being approximately 12 hours.

Elimination. The drug is metabolized in the liver and excreted in the urine and feces.

Uses

Loxapine is used in the treatment of psychotic disorders. Loxapine appears to be as effective as the other neuroleptics.

Cautions

In general, the same precautions associated with the use of PTZs applies to loxapine, despite the fact that it is chemically different from the PTZs and that some side effects have been reported with PTZs which have not yet been reported to occur with loxapine. (See the section on PTZs for details.) Most side effects appear to be dose-related. Drowsiness is a common initial side effect. In general, expyramidal symptoms respond well to anticholinergic medications. Tardive dyskinesia and NMS may occur with use of loxapine. Loxapine has anticholinergic effects. Furthermore, adverse cardiovascular effects may include hypotension and tachycardia. Loxapine may cause photosensitivity. Patients should be cautioned that loxapine may impair mental alertness and physical coordination and that activities which require these abilities should be engaged in with caution. The drug should be used with caution in patients with a history of seizure disorder.

Indications and efficacy have not been established for the use of loxapine in children younger than 16 years of age.

Toxicity

Manifestations. Overdosage with loxapine presents as an extension of the underlying side effects. Associated with this are seizures and CNS depression which may progress to coma. Treatment consists of supportive therapy and removal of the drug by gastric lavage if possible. Seizures may be controlled with benzodiazepines or barbiturates; extrapyramidal reactions may be controlled with anticholinergic or antiparkinsonian agents, and severe hypotension may be treated with norepinephrine or phenylephrine.

Dosage and Administration

Dosage. Loxapine 15 mg is the therapeutic equivalent of 2 mg of haloperidol. The usual initial oral adult dosage is 10 mg twice a day. This may be increased as tolerated and needed. For severe psychosis an initial oral dose of 50 mg/day is common. Usual maintenance is 60 to 100 mg/day administered in 2 to 4 divided doses. In general, oral dosage should not exceed 250 mg/day. The usual initial IM dosage is 12.5 to 50 mg every 4 to 6 hours as indicated; dosage is adjusted as needed.

Administration. Loxapine succinate is administered orally; loxapine hydrochloride is administered by IM injection or orally. IM administration is used for acutely agitated patients or those in whom oral administration is not possible. Loxapine oral concentrate solution should be diluted prior to administration.

Preparations

Loxapine hydrochloride
- Oral solution, concentrate (*Loxitane C oral concentrate*)
  - 25 mg/mL

Loxapine succinate
- Parenteral injection (*Loxitane IM*)
  - 50 mg/mL
- Oral capsules (*Loxitane*)
  - 5 mg, 10 mg, 25 mg, 50 mg

MESORIDAZINE BESYLATE

Chemical Class: Piperidine Phenothiazine

Pharmacology

The principle pharmacologic effects of mesoridazine are similar to those of thioridazine. Mesoridazine has moderate anticholinergic effects, weak extrapyramidal effects, weak antiemetic effects, and strong sedative effects.

Pharmacokinetics

Mesoridazine is well absorbed from the GI tract following oral administration and has a half-life of approximately 24 to 48 hours. Mesoridazine and its metabolites are excreted in the urine and feces.

Uses

Mesoridazine is used for the symptomatic control of psychotic disorders. In general, this drug, like other neuroleptics, is effective in reducing conceptual disorganization, anxiety, hallucinations, suspiciousness, and emotional withdrawal.

Cautions

Mesoridazine shares the cautions associated with other PTZs. (See the General Statement regarding PTZs for details.) Drowsiness and hypotension are the most frequent adverse effects with mesoridazine. In children younger than 12 years of age, the safety and efficacy of mesoridazine have not been established.

Dosage and Administration

Dosage. Mesoridazine 50 mg is the therapeutic equivalent of 2 mg of haloperidol. Dosage must be titrated to the individual's need and tolerance. Lower doses are used in the young and geriatric age groups. Those patients receiving long-term therapy should be periodically reevaluated for continued indication and for the development of adverse side effects. Initial dosage is usually 50 mg three times a day. Many psychotic patients are treated effectively with 100 to 400 mg/day. Patients with organic brain syndromes or mental retardation may need lower doses than those typically used in adult populations. The usual initial adult dosage of mesoridazine for IM preparations is 25 mg. Maximum IM dosage in adults usually does not exceed 400 mg/day.

Administration. Mesoridazine besylate is administered orally or by deep IM injection. The oral concentrate must be diluted before use.

Preparations

Mesoridazine besylate (*Serentil*)
- Oral solution, concentrate
  - 25 mg/mL
- Tablets
  - 10 mg, 25 mg, 50 mg, 100 mg

Parenteral injection
25 mg/mL

MOLINDONE HYDROCHLORIDE

Chemical Class: Dihydroindolone

Pharmacology

The pharmacologic effect of molindone is similar to that of the phenothiazines. It is moderately sedating, with mild antiadrenergic, anticholinergic, and extrapyramidal effects. Many practitioners believe that molindone has a lower frequency of weight gain, as an adverse effect, than the other neuroleptics.

Pharmacokinetics

Molindone is rapidly absorbed from the GI tract with peak plasma concentrations occurring in approximately 1 hour. Molindone is metabolized in the liver and excreted in the urine and feces. Less than 3% of the unmetabolized drug is excreted.

Uses

Molindone is used in the treatment of psychosis and appears to be as effective as the PTZs. Individual responses to antipsychotic drugs are, however, highly variable.

Cautions

Adverse Effects. The toxic manifestations of molindone resemble those of the PTZs. (See the General Statement regarding PTZs for details.) Drowsiness is a frequent side effect. Extrapyramidal syndromes are usually dose-related and may be controlled with either an anticholinergic antiparkinsonian drug, or by modification of the administered dose. More serious consequences of molindone administration include tardive dyskinesia and NMS. Molindone may have adverse effects on the autonomic nervous system, including nasal congestion, constipation, dry mouth, and blurred vision. There may also be dizziness, headache, nausea, anorexia, and GI upset. Tachycardia, postural hypotension, weight change, and hypothermia may occur. Lactation or gynecomastia have occurred infrequently.

Precautions and Contraindications

The profile of toxic side effects associated with molindone is similar to that of other antipsychotic agents. (See the General

Statement regarding PTZs for details.) Molindone may impair physical coordination or mental alertness. For this reason, patients should be cautioned about engaging in activities which require such abilities.

Some preparations of molindone hydrochloride contain sodium metabisulfite. This may cause allergic-type reactions, including life-threatening asthmatic responses and anaphylaxis in susceptible individuals. The overall incidence of sulfite sensitivity is highest in asthmatic individuals. The safety and efficacy of molindone therapy in children younger than 12 years of age have not been established.

Acute toxic manifestations of overdose represent an extension of the usual toxic side effects. There are severe extrapyramidal reactions and sedation. A shocklike syndrome may occur. There may be respiratory depression. Severe hypotension is associated with the shocklike syndrome. Supportive therapy is indicated. Early gastric lavage may be helpful in removing drugs. Anticholinergic, antiparkinsonian agents may be used to treat severe extrapyramidal reactions. Peritoneal and hemodialysis are ineffective in the removal of molindone. Charcoal administration, especially during the first 24 hours, may help decrease GI absorption.

Dosage and Administration

Dosage. Molindone 10 mg is the therapeutic equivalent of 2 mg of haloperidol. Dosage must be titrated to the most effective dose for maintenance therapy. Initial therapy should be titrated to the patient's needs and tolerance. Geriatric and debilitated patients are usually started on lower doses than young adults. The usual starting adult dosage of molindone hydrochloride is 50 to 75 mg/day, in divided doses. This may be increased up to 225 mg if needed. In cases of mild psychosis, 5 to 15 mg, administered 3 or 4 times a day, is often adequate. Often, with moderately severe symptomatology, 10 to 25 mg, three to four times a day, is administered. Many clinicians believe that dosages greater than 150 mg/day rarely produce additional clinical benefit.

Administration. Molindone hydrochloride is administered orally.

Preparations

Molindone hydrochloride (*Moban*)
  Oral solution
    20 mg/mL

Tablets

5 mg, 10 mg, 25 mg, 50 mg, 100 mg

PERPHENAZINE

Chemical Class: Piperazine Phenothiazine

Pharmacology

The pharmacologic effects of perphenazine are similar to those of chlorpromazine. Perphenazine has strong antiemetic activity, moderate to strong extrapyramidal effects, mild to moderate anticholinergic and antiadrenergic effects, and moderate sedative effects.

Pharmacokinetics

Perphenazine is readily absorbed from GI tract and metabolized by hepatic enzymes before excretion in urine and feces.

Uses

Perphenazine is used for the management of psychotic disorders. The patient response to antipsychotic drugs is variable, and those patients who do not respond adequately to perphenazine should be tried with a different therapeutic agent.

Cautions

The precautions associated with PTZ use in general should be observed. (See the General Statement regarding PTZs for details.) Some preparations of perphenazine contain sodium bisulfite. This may cause allergic-type reactions including severe asthmatic episodes and anaphylaxis. Sulfite sensitivity is more common in asthmatic individuals.

Dosage and Administration

Dosage. Perphenazine 10 mg is the therapeutic equivalent of 2 mg of haloperidol. Dosage must be titrated to the individual's needs and tolerance. For moderately disturbed outpatients, the usual initial dosage of perphenazine in adults and children over 12 years of age is 4 to 8 mg, three times a day. In hospitalized adults and adolescents, the usual initial oral dose is 8 to 16 mg, 2 to 4 times per day. In most cases the oral dosage of perphenazine should not exceed 64 mg/day. When oral therapy is not possible or when prompt control of severe symptoms is required, parenteral administration may be indicated. The usual initial IM dose of perphenazine is 5 mg. This may be repeated every 6 hours as needed. In severely agitated patients the initial dosage may be 10 mg. The IM dosage of perphenazine generally should not exceed 30 mg/day.

Administration. Perphenazine is most commonly administered orally; however, it may be administered by deep IM injection or by IV infusion. The oral concentrate solution must be diluted prior to use. During IV administration blood pressure and pulse must be monitored continuously in an environment with supportive equipment and drugs for the management of acute hypotensive episodes or severe extrapyramidal reactions.

Preparations

Perphenazine (*Trilafon*)
- Oral solution, concentrate
  - 16 mg/5 mL
- Tablets
  - 2 mg, 4 mg, 8 mg, 16 mg
- Parenteral injection
  - 5 mg/mL

Perphenazine and amitriptyline hydrochloride
- Oral tablets
  - 2 mg perphenazine and 10 mg amitriptyline hydrochloride (*Etrafon 2-10*)
  - 2 mg perphenazine and 25 mg amitriptyline hydrochloride (*Etrafon*)
  - 4 mg perphenazine and 10 mg amitriptylinhydrochloride (*Etrafon A*)
  - 4 mg perphenazine and 25 mg amitriptyline hydrochloride (*Etrafon Forte* tablets, film-coated)
  - 2 mg perphenazine and 10 mg amitriptyline hydrochloride (*Triavil 2-10*)
  - 2 mg perphenazine and 25 mg amitriptyline hydrochloride (*Triavil 2-25*)
  - 4 mg perphenazine and 10 mg amitriptyline hydrochloride (*Triavil 4-10*)
  - 4 mg perphenazine and 25 mg amitriptyline hydrochloride (*Triavil 4-25*)
  - 4 mg perphenazine and 50 mg amitriptyline hydrochloride (*Triavil 4-50*)

PIMOZIDE

Chemical Class: Diphenylbutylpiperidine

Pharmacology

The effects of pimozide are similar to those of haloperidol and, to a degree, the PTZs. Pimozide has weak anticholinergic, antiadrenergic, and sedative effects, but strong extrapyramidal effects.
The D_2 receptor antagonist properties of pimozide are thought to be the mechanism behind its ability to suppress motor and vocal tics in Gilles de la Tourette's syndrome. This D_2 blockade is also thought to explain its antipsychotic action. D_2 receptor antagonism occurs predominantly on postsynaptic receptor sites, although to a lesser degree there is some blockade of presynaptic D_2 sites. Pimozide has not been shown to have a significant effect on other catecholamines. Pimozide may lower the seizure threshold, and it may produce an increase in alpha wave activity on the EEG.

Pimozide is an antiemetic. This is mediated via a direct effect on the chemoreceptor trigger zone. The drug also has weak antispasmodic effects.

Pharmacokinetics

Absorption. Pimozide is absorbed slowly from the GI tract. Peak plasma concentration of the drug occurs within about 6 hours of administration. There is considerable individual variation in drug absorption and peak plasma levels.

Distribution. The distribution of pimozide in the body has not been well described. It is known, however, that the highest concentrations in the brain occur in the caudate nucleus and the pituitary.

Elimination. The steady-state elimination half-life is approximately 55 hours. There is a wide variation in this figure. The drug undergoes extensive first-pass metabolism. It is metabolized by oxidative N-dealkylation in the liver. It is unknown if the metabolites possess pharmacologic activity in man. Pimozide and its metabolites are excreted principally in the urine.

Uses

Gilles de la Tourette's syndrome. The motor and vocal tics of Gilles de la Tourette's syndrome can be suppressed with pimozide. Pimozide is considered a first-line agent in the treatment of this disorder. It is only used in those who have vocal and motor tics severe enough to compromise their function in daily life. It should not be used for the suppression of mild or minor tics.

Some studies suggest that pimozide may be as effective as haloperidol in the management of Gilles de la Tourette's syndrome. Its use may be associated with less severe and possibly less frequent adverse effects. The long-term safety of pimozide has not been determined.

Other Uses. Pimozide has been used in the management of chronic schizophrenia. In general, however, other neuroleptics are more commonly used. It does appear to be as effective as the PTZs in the management of chronic schizophrenia. Pimozide has also been used in the treatment of the acute stage of schizophrenia, though studies suggest that higher doses may be necessary. Higher doses are associated with a higher incidence and severity of extrapyramidal reactions. Pimozide has also been used in the treatment of acute mania, and may be as effective as PTZs in this population. It has also been used to treat a variety of other conditions, such as various personality disorders, phencyclidine-induced psychosis, and erotomania.

Pimozide may reduce irritability, anxiety, hyperactivity, and mental retardation. It may also improve social behavior in mentally retarded adolescents. There does not appear to be a substantial negative impact on cognition or learning performance with this drug.

Cautions

Extrapyramidal Reactions. Extrapyramidal reactions occur frequently during the initial treatment with pimozide. The reactions are usually dose-dependent, and they disappear with discontinuation of the drug. Most commonly, tremor, rigidity, and akinesia occur. The incidence has been estimated at 10% to 15% of those patients exposed to pimozide. Frequently, extrapyramidal reactions will respond to the administration of either diphenhydramine, or anticholinergic, antiparkinsonian agents such as benztropine or trihexyphenidyl.

Dystonic reactions may occur; torticollis may be especially frequent. There may be accompanying orofacial symptoms and less commonly an oculogyric crisis. Pimozide has been associated with akathisia. This is usually managed by either dose reduction or the administration of an anticholinergic, antiparkinsonian agent; diphenhydramine; a benzodiazepine; or propranolol. Pimozide has also been associated with the development of NMS. (See the General Statement regarding PTZs for details on NMS.)

Tardive Dyskinesia. Pimozide has been associated with the development of tardive dyskinesia. (See the General Statement regarding PTZ for details regarding tardive dyskinesia.)

Other Nervous System Effects. The most common adverse effects associated with pimozide are sedation, lethargy, and drowsiness. Anticholinergic effects are associated with pimozide and include dry mouth, constipation, urinary retention, blurred vision, and memory impairment.

Cardiovascular Effects. Pimozide has been associated with orthostatic hypotension, tachycardia, and palpitations. It is also associated with prolongation of the QT interval; flattening, notching, and inversion of the T wave; and the development of U waves. The clinical significance of these changes is unclear. It is unknown if prolongation of the QT interval predisposes these patients to ventricular arrhythmia. Patients should be screened with a baseline ECG prior to the administration of pimozide. During treatment with pimozide, an ECG should then be re-obtained if clinical evidence suggests cardiac dysrhythmia or bundle-branch block.

Endocrine and Metabolic Effects. Mild galactorrhea, dysmenorrhea, and amenorrhea have been reported to occur with pimozide. Pimozide increases serum prolactin concentration.

Other Adverse Effects. Rash, urticaria, skin irritation, and edema may occur. Patients may be unusually sensitive to light.

Cautions

See the General Statement regarding PTZs for a discussion of the general toxic potential of antipsychotic drugs. As with all such drugs, an informed decision should be made about the risks vs. benefits prior to the administration of the drug and prior to placing the patient on a long-term course with this agent. Patients and, if applicable, their family or guardians should be informed about the long-term risk of tardive dyskinesia.

Data on the use and efficacy of pimozide in children younger than 12 years of age are limited. The safety and efficacy of pimozide for the treatment of conditions other than Gilles de la Tourette's syndrome in children have not been evaluated.

Dosage and Administration

Dosage. For symptomatic treatment in Gilles de la Tourette's syndrome, the initial dosage should be low and gradually titrated upward if needed. The patient should have an ECG performed prior to administration of the drug. The usual initial dose for treatment of Gilles de la Tourette's syndrome is 1 to 2 mg/day. This may be increased every other day as tolerated. Dosage is usually increased in 1-mg increments and increased until limited either by side effects or until a therapeutic response occurs. Most patients respond with dosages of less than 0.2 mg/kg/day or 10 mg/day, whichever is less. As with all neuroleptics the lowest clinically effective dose should be administered. Attempts at dose reduction should be made every 6 to 12 months after successful treatment has been achieved. Reduction in dosage should occur gradually in all cases of dose reduction or discontinuation of pimozide.

Administration. Pimozide is administered orally, and it may be administered either in divided doses or once a day.

Preparations

Pimozide (*Orap*)
Oral tablets
2 mg

PROCHLORPERAZINE, PROCHLORPERAZINE EDISYLATE, PROCHLORPERAZINE MALEATE

Chemical Class: Piperazine Phenothiazine

Pharmacology

The pharmacologic actions of prochlorperazine are similar to those of CPZ. Prochlorperazine has strong antiemetic activity, strong extrapyramidal effects, and moderate sedative and weak anticholinergic effects.

Pharmacokinetics

Prochlorperazine is readily absorbed from the GI tract after oral or rectal administration. It is partially absorbed from IM injection sites. Hepatic metabolites are excreted in urine and feces.

Uses

Prochlorperazine is primarily used as an antiemetic and rarely used to treat psychotic disorders. Patient response to antipsychotic agents is variable, and those individuals who do not adequately respond to one antipsychotic should be given trials with other agents.

Cautions

Prochlorperazine shares the toxic potential of other PTZ antipsychotics. (See the General Statement on PTZs for a review of toxicity.) The incidence of extrapyramidal reactions appears to be high in prochlorperazine therapy. Therefore, the clinician needs to be alert to the possibility of akathisia or other extrapyramidal side effects, even in those patients who are receiving the drug as an antiemetic. Some preparations contain sulfites which may cause allergic-type reactions in susceptible individuals, including anaphylaxis and severe asthmatic episodes. While the overall prevalence of sulfite sensitivity in the general population is low, such sensitivity is more common in asthmatic individuals.

Dosage and Administration

Dosage. Prochlorperazine 15 mg is the therapeutic equivalent of 2 mg of haloperidol. Dosage must be titrated to the individual's need and tolerance. The lowest possible effective dose should be used. Those patients receiving the IM preparation should be converted to oral preparations as soon as clinically possible. Lower dosages should be used in adolescents and in geriatric patients. Adverse effects are more common with long-term administration. Those patients receiving long-term neuroleptics should be reexamined for continued indications for administration and to assess the possible development of adverse side effects. For outpatient treatment of mild psychotic symptomatology, the usual adult dosage of prochlorperazine is 5 to 10 mg 3 to 4 times a day. For hospitalized patients with moderate to severe symptoms the usual initial dosage is 10 mg 3 to 4 times a day. Dosage is gradually increased until symptoms are controlled. Many patients are adequately controlled with 50 to 75 mg/day, but, some patients may require dosages up to 150 mg/day. The initial oral or rectal dosage of prochlorperazine in children aged 2 to 12 years is 2.5 mg 2 to 3 times a day. Dosage generally does not exceed 20 mg/day in children 2 to 5 years of age, and 25 mg/day in children 6 to 12 years of age.

The usual IM dose of prochlorperazine is 10 to 20 mg. This may be repeated every 4 to 6 hours. In children older than 12 years, the usual IM dose is 0.13 mg/kg. The extended-release preparations (Spansule) may be administered once every 12 hours.

Nausea and Vomiting. For antiemetic purposes the usual recommended dose is 5 to 10 mg, orally or IM, every 4 to 6 hours; or 25 mg, rectally, twice daily.

Administration. Prochlorperazine maleate is administered orally. Prochlorperazine is administered rectally. Prochlorperazine edisylate is administered by IV injection or IV infusion and is used in the treatment of severe nausea and vomiting. Prochlorperazine edisylate is administered orally or by IM injection for psychiatric use.

Preparations

Prochlorperazine (*Compazine*)
- Rectal suppositories
  - 2.5 mg, 5.0 mg, 25 mg

Prochlorperazine edisylate
- Oral solution (*Compazine Syrup*)
  - 5 mg/mL
- Parenteral injection (*Compazine*)
  - 5 mg/mL

Prochlorperazine maleate
- Oral capsules, extended-release (*Compazine, Spansule*)
  - 10 mg, 15 mg, 30 mg
- Tablets, film-coated (*Compazine*)
  - 5 mg, 10 mg, 25 mg

PROMAZINE HYDROCHLORIDE

Chemical Class: Aliphatic Phenothiazine

Pharmacology

The general pharmacologic effects of promazine are similar to those of CPZ. Promazine is less potent on a weight basis than CPZ. It has strong anticholinergic and sedative effects, moderate extrapyramidal effects, moderate antiemetic activity, weak antipsychotic activity, and it is not commonly used. Promazine is used principally as an antiemetic, especially for postoperative nausea and vomiting.

Pharmacokinetics

Promazine is readily absorbed from the GI tract. Hepatic metabolites are excreted in urine and feces.

Uses

Promazine is used for the control of psychotic disorders. Patient response to PTZ antipsychotics is variable. Those patients who do not respond adequately to one PTZ should be tried on other agents. It should be noted, however, that promazine has weak antipsychotic activity.

Cautions

Promazine shares the toxic potentials of other PTZ antipsychotic agents. (See the General Statement on PTZs for details.) Those most frequent adverse effects are drowsiness and orthostatic hypotension. *Sparine* 25-mg tablets contain tartrazine (FD&C yellow no. 5) which may produce an allergic reaction, including bronchial asthma, in susceptible individuals. Susceptibility occurs most commonly in patients who are sensitive to aspirin. In addition, some preparations contain sulfites. These may cause allergic-type reactions including anaphylaxis or severe asthmatic episodes in susceptible individuals. Susceptibility appears to occur more commonly in asthmatic individuals. The safety and efficacy of promazine have not been established in children younger than 12 years.

Dosage and Administration

Dosage. The oral and IM dosages of promazine hydrochloride are the same. The usual oral or IM dose for the management of psychotic disorders is 10 to 200 mg every 4 to 6 hours. Dosages up to 800 mg have been used in some adults. Single oral dosages of 500 mg have been well tolerated. It is recommended that the daily total dose not exceed 1 g since higher doses do not increase the general positive effects. The incidence of adverse effects increases with a long-term administration of the drug. For this reason, patients on chronic therapy should be periodically reevaluated both for development of toxic side effects and for continued indications for drug treatment.

Nausea and Vomiting. For antiemesis the usual dose is 25 to 50 mg, orally or IM, every 4 to 6 hours.

Administration. Promazine is usually administered orally. It may also be administered by IM injection or IV injection. IM injections may produce significant hypotension and local irritation. If IM administration is required, many practitioners prefer to use high-potency neuroleptics. If parenteral treatment is used, patients should be kept in a recumbent position.

Preparation

Promazine hydrochloride
- Oral tablets
  - 25 mg, 50 mg, 100 mg (*Sparine*)
- Parenteral injection
  - 25 mg/mL (*Promazine hydrochloride injection*)
  - 50 mg/mL (*Promazine-50, Sparine*)

RISPERIDONE

Risperidone represents a significant advance in the treatment of schizophrenia.

Pharmacology

Risperidone is chemically unrelated to other available antipsychotics. It is believed to exert its therapeutic effects in schizophrenia by blocking dopaminergic and serotonergic receptors. It is also an antagonist of alpha-adrenergic and histaminergic receptors. The antidopaminergic properties may be responsible for its effects on positive symptoms of schizophrenia. The serotonin blocking effects may account for its efficacy in treating negative symptoms of schizophrenia. This unique pharmacologic profile is also responsible for risperidone's ability to be an effective antipsychotic with a low incidence of side effects.

Pharmacokinetics

Absorption. The bioavailability of risperidone is approximately 70%. Food does not affect the absorption of risperidone. Thus, it can be given with or without meals.

Metabolism. Risperidone is metabolized to an active metabolite, 9-hydroxyrisperidone (9-HR). This metabolite appears to be as effective as risperidone at binding to receptors. Thus, both compounds probably exert antipsychotic effects in patients.

Distribution. Approximately 90% of risperidone and 75% of 9-HR are bound to serum proteins. Peak serum levels of the parent compound are achieved approximately 1 hour after ingestion. Rapid metabolizers of risperidone reach peak 9-HR levels in approximately 3 hours. Slow metabolizers reach peak 9-HR levels by up to 17 hours.

Elimination. Risperidone has a half-life of approximately 3 hours in rapid metabolizers and 20 hours in poor metabolizers. Thus, patients may reach steady-state levels of risperidone anywhere between 1–5 days, depending on how rapidly the drug is metabolized. Steady-state of the metabolite is reached in 5–6 days.

Clearance of risperidone in patients with renal disease is 60% lower than in healthy subjects.

In liver diseases, the pharmacokinetics of risperidone do not change, but the free drug available in such patients can be increased by 35% due to reduced serum binding proteins.

As expected, elderly patients clear risperidone more slowly and accumulate higher steady-state levels than do young controls.

Uses

Risperidone is a highly effective antipsychotic drug used for the treatment of psychosis, for which it is approved in this country. It is at least as effective as other antipsychotics currently available in the U.S. In many patients, it may be more effective than most antipsychotic medications, particularly in the treatment of negative symptoms of schizophrenia. Some evidence suggests that it is effective for patients who are nonpartial responders to other classes of antipsychotics.

Cautions

Adverse Effects. In phase 2 and 3 trials, 9% of risperidone-treated patients discontinued treatment because of adverse effects. This is contrasted with the 7% of patients on placebo and 10% of patients on other antipsychotics who stopped treatment because of adverse effects in those trials.

Risperidone can produce orthostatic hypotension and reflex tachycardia, presumably due to blockade of alpha-adrenergic receptors. However, slow upward titration of doses appears to significantly minimize this complication.

Tardive dyskinesia (TD), an involuntary dyskinetic disorder often involving the facial musculature, can develop in patients on antipsychotics. The actual incidence of TD due to risperidone is unclear. Some have suggested that risperidone may produce TD less often than in older antipsychotics. However, large long-term studies are needed to substantiate these claims.

Some patients experience QT prolongation with risperidone.

Like most other antipsychotics, risperidone can cause weight gain and elevation of serum prolactin levels. Unlike clozapine, risperidone does not appear to produce adverse hematologic effects. Therefore, frequent CBC monitoring is not indicated in risperidone-treated patients.

The most common adverse effects of risperidone are insomnia (25% of patients), agitation (25%), EPS (17%–34% depending on dosage), and anxiety (15%). Interestingly, at the standard dose of 6 mg each day, the incidence of EPS was no higher in treated patients than in placebo-treated subjects. Given that EPS side effects are a major reason patients discontinue antipsychotics, risperidone may be associated with better compliance than other antipsychotics.

Precautions and Contraindications

Caution should be used in geriatric patients and in patients with hepatic or renal dysfunction. A lower dose should be used in these patients. Patients should be advised of the risk of hypotension, especially during the period of initial dose titration.

Toxicity

There are rare to infrequent reports of overdose with risperidone. One subject who took an overdose experienced hyponatremia, hypokalemia, and prolongation of QT and QRS on EKG. One overdose was associated with a seizure. There have been no fatalities or permanent sequelae described. Symptoms of overdose included drowsiness, hypotension, tachycardia, and extrapyramidal symptoms. Gastric lavage and activated charcoal may help reduce the sequelae of an overdose. General supportive measures should be undertaken with concurrent cardiac and vital signs monitoring.

Drug Interactions

Because of its alpha-adrenergic blockade with subsequent postural hypotension, risperidone may enhance the effects of other drugs lowering blood pressure. Risperidone may antagonize the effects of dopamine agonists. Chronic administration of clozapine with risperidone may reduce clearance of risperidone. However, chronic administration of carbamazepine may increase clearance of risperidone.

Dosage and Administration

The manufacturer recommends twice-a-day dosing, although some believe that a single daily dose of risperidone can be safe and effective. Dosing of risperidone can begin at 1 mg bid. This may be increased within a few days to 3 mg bid. In some patients, slower titration may be required. The drug is substantially superior to placebo for chronic schizophrenia in doses from 4 to 16 mg per day. However, 6 mg per day appears to produce the optimal therapeutic effect for most adult patients. Patients with renal or hepatic disease should receive lower doses. Some recommend geriatric patients be given one-half the dose of other populations. Some evidence suggests that doses as low as 0.25 mg bid are effective for elderly patients. The recommended initial dose is 0.5 mg bid in patients who are elderly or debilitated, patients with severe renal or hepatic impairment, and patients either predisposed to hypotension or for whom hypotension would pose a risk. Dosage increases in these patients should be in increments of no more than 0.5 mg bid. Increases to dosages above 1.5 mg bid should generally occur at intervals of at least 1 week. In some patients, slower titration may be medically appropriate.

Switching from another antipsychotic to risperidone should be done so as to involve as little overlap between the two drugs as possible.

Administration. Risperidone is administered orally.

Preparations

Risperidone (*Risperdal*)
  Oral tablets
    1 mg (scored), 2 mg, 3 mg, 4 mg

THIORIDAZINE, THIORIDAZINE HYDROCHLORIDE

Chemical Class: Piperidine Phenothiazine

Pharmacology

The general pharmacologic effects of thioridazine are similar to those of chlorpromazine. On a weight basis thioridazine is about as potent as chlorpromazine. It has strong antiadrenergic, anticholinergic, and sedative effects, with weak extrapyramidal and antiemetic activity.

Pharmacokinetics

Thioridazine is variably absorbed from the GI tract. Hepatic metabolism produces metabolites that are excreted in the urine and feces. One of the metabolites, mesoridazine, may account for most of the clinical efficacy of thioridazine.

Uses

Thioridazine is used in the management of acute psychotic disorders. Patient response to PTZ antipsychotics is variable. Individuals who do not respond to one drug should be tried with other agents. The lowest effective dose should be used. Those patients on long-term therapy should receive periodic examinations for the assessment of potential toxic side effects and to assess indication for continued use.

Cautions

Thioridazine shares the general toxic potentials of other PTZs. (See the General Statement on PTZs for details.) Pigmentary retinopathy is a significant risk at doses greater than 500 mg/day; therefore 800 mg/day should be considered an absolute dose limit. Inhibition of ejaculation, retrograde ejaculation, and ECG changes may all occur more frequently with thioridazine than with other neuroleptics.

Dosage and Administration

Dosage. Thioridazine 100 mg is the therapeutic equivalent of 2 mg of haloperidol. Dosage must be titrated to the individual's tolerance and needs. The usual initial dose is 50 to 100 mg three times a day. Dosage may be titrated up to 800 mg/day given in 2 to 4 divided doses. Dosages greater than 300 mg are usually reserved for severe neuropsychiatric conditions. For children between 2 and 12 years of age the usual dosage is 0.5 to 3.0 mg/kg/day. Dosages for children under 2 years of age have not been established.

Administration. Thioridazine and thioridazine hydrochloride are administered orally. The oral concentrate should be diluted before administration.

Preparations

Thioridazine

Oral suspension (*Mellaril-S*)

25 mg/5 mL, 100 mg/5 mL

Oral solution, concentrate

(*Mellaril Concentrate,Thioridazine HCI Intensol*)

30 mg/mL, 100 mg/mL

Tablets (*Mellaril*)

10 mg, 15 mg, 25 mg, 50 mg, 100 mg, 150 mg, 200 mg

THIOTHIXENE, THIOTHIXENE HYDROCHLORIDE
Chemical Class: Thioxanthene

Pharmacology

The pharmacologic action of thiothixene is similar to that of piperazine PTZs. Thiothixene has weak sedative, anticholinergic, and antiadrenergic effects, with strong extrapyramidal effects.

Pharmacokinetics

Absorption. Thiothixene is rapidly absorbed from the GI tract. It is also well absorbed following parenteral injection.

Distribution. Thiothixene is widely distributed in body tissues.

Elimination. Thiothixene is metabolized in the liver and excreted mainly in the feces.

Uses

Thiothixene is used in the treatment of psychosis. Like other neuroleptics it appears to be more effective in ameliorating the positive symptoms associated with schizophrenia rather than the negative symptoms.

Cautions

Adverse Effects. The adverse effects associated with thiothixene are similar to those seen with all neuroleptics. (See the General Statement regarding PTZs for details.) Side effects are usually dose-dependent. Common side effects associated with thiothixene are extrapyramidal symptoms and drowsiness. It may also produce akathisia and dystonia. Extrapyramidal effects respond well to anticholinergic, antiparkinsonian agents. Tardive dyskinesia may develop after prolonged administration. Thiothixene has a variety of effects on the autonomic nervous system. These include dry mouth, blurred vision, constipation, diaphoresis, salivation, and impotence. Thiothixene has been associated with nonspecific ECG changes. It is unclear whether these are of clinical importance. They are reversible and disappear with discontinuation of drug therapy. Hypotension may occur following parenteral administration. Thiothixene may produce drowsiness, fatigue, ataxia, and syncope. For this reason, patients should be cautioned about performing hazardous tasks such as those requiring mental alertness or physical coordination. Thiothixene should be administered with caution to those patients with a history of seizure disorder since the drug may decrease the seizure threshold.

Thiothixene may produce pigmentary retinopathy and lenticular pigmentation. For this reason patients should receive periodic slit-lamp examinations if they are receiving prolonged thiothixene therapy.

Pediatric Precautions. Because of limited data this drug should be used with caution in children younger than 12 years of age. Thiothixene has not been demonstrated to have clinical efficacy in that age group.

Toxicity

Manifestations. Overdose may produce hypotension, ataxia, rigidity, weakness, tremor, torticollis, and dysphagia. This may progress to CNS depression including coma.

Treatment. Primary treatment consists of supportive measures such as maintenance of an adequate airway and prevention of circulatory collapse. Early in overdose, gastric lavage and charcoal administration may be helpful. Epinephrine should not be used for the maintenance of circulation. Thiothixene causes a reversal of its vasopressor effects and a further lowering of blood pressure. For this reason norepinephrine or phenylephrine should be used.

Drug Interactions

There may be additive effects between thiothixene and other CNS depressants such as alcohol, anticholinergics, or hypotensive agents. Thiothixene may potentiate the hypotensive effects of agents used in the control of hypertension.

Dosage and Administration

Dosage. Thiothixene 4 mg is the therapeutic equivalent of 2 mg of haloperidol. The usual adult dosage for mild psychosis is 2 mg three times a day. Dosage may be increased up to 15 mg/day. In cases of severe psychosis the initial therapy may be 5 mg twice a day with subsequent upward titration to 20 to 30 mg/day. Dosages as high as 60 mg/day have been used. Beyond this level there is usually no further therapeutic benefit, but there is a further development of side effects. The usual initial adult IM dose in acutely agitated patients is 4 mg 2 to 4 times a day. This may be increased further as needed to 16 to 20 mg/day. The usual IM dose does not exceed 30 mg/day. After adequate clinical control has been obtained, most patients are switched to oral agents as soon as possible.

Administration. Thiothixene is administered orally. Thiothixene hydrochloride is administered orally or by IM injection.

Preparations

Thiothixene
- Oral capsules (*Navane*)
  - 1 mg, 2 mg, 5 mg, 10 mg, 20 mg

Thiothixene hydrochloride
- Oral solution (*Navane Concentrate*)
  - 5 mg/mL
- Parenteral injection, for IM use (*Navane Intramuscular*)
  - 10 mg

TRIFLUOPERAZINE HYDROCHLORIDE

Chemical Class: Piperazine Phenothiazine

Pharmacology

Trifluoperazine hydrochloride has similar actions to CPZ. It has strong antiemetic activity and strong extrapyramidal effects. It has weak anticholinergic effects and antiadrenergic effects, with weak to moderate sedative effects. Trifluoperazine has a longer duration of action than CPZ and greater potency on a weight basis.

Pharmacokinetics

Trifluoperazine is readily absorbed from the GI tract and parenteral injection sites. Hepatic metabolites are excreted in the urine and feces.

Uses

Trifluoperazine is used to treat psychotic disorders. Some patients may preferentially respond to one psychotropic as opposed to another. For this reason, when patients fail to adequately respond to trifluoperazine they should be treated with other neuroleptics.

Cautions

Trifluoperazine shares the toxic potential of other PTZ antipsychotic agents. (See the General Statement regarding PTZs for details.) Trifluoperazine produces a high incidence of extrapyramidal reactions. Piperazine compounds are preferred among the PTZs for patients with cardiovascular disease, since no significant ECG changes have been noted.

Dosage and Administration

Dosage. Trifluoperazine 5 mg is the therapeutic equivalent of 2 mg of haloperidol. Dosage must be titrated to the lowest effective dose. Because the risk for adverse side effects increases with prolonged use of the drug, patients receiving this drug on a chronic basis should be periodically reevaluated for the development of toxic side effects and for continued indications for treatment. Lower dosages should be used in the geriatric population. Maximum response usually occurs after 2 to 3 weeks of administration. For outpatients the usual initial dose is 1 to 2 mg twice a day with dosage seldom exceeding 4 mg/day. For more severely ill patients, the initial dose is 2 to 5 mg twice a day with most patients having a therapeutic response between 15 and 20 mg/day. In general, doses exceeding 40 mg/day are rarely indicated. The usual dose for severely ill children aged 6 to 12 years is 1 mg once or twice a day. This is titrated upward as needed with dosage seldom exceeding 15 mg/day. The indications for use of trifluoperazine in children younger than 6 years of age have not been established.

The usual IM dose is 1 to 2 mg every 4 to 6 hours, adjusted as necessary. Dosages rarely exceed 10 mg IM in 24 hours.

Administration. Trifluoperazine hydrochloride is administered orally in most cases. IM administration is reserved for when oral therapy is not possible. The oral concentrate needs dilution prior to administration.

Preparations

Trifluoperazine hydrochloride
  Oral solution, concentrate (*Stelazine Concentrate*)
    10 mg/mL
  Tablets (*Stelazine*)
    1 mg, 2 mg, 5 mg, 10 mg
  Parenteral injection (*Stelazine*)
    2 mg/mL

TRIFLUPROMAZINE

Chemical Class: Aliphatic Phenothiazine

Pharmacology

The pharmacologic effects of triflupromazine are similar to those of the PTZs. (See the General Statement regarding PTZs for details.) This compound has strong anticholinergic and antiadrenergic effects with moderate to strong sedative and extrapyramidal effects.

Pharmacokinetics

Triflupromazine is readily absorbed from IM injection sites. Products of hepatic metabolism are excreted in urine and feces.

Uses

Triflupromazine is used for the management of psychosis. It is also used as an antiemetic.

Cautions

The side effect profile of triflupromazine is similar to that of the PTZs. (See the General Statement regarding PTZs for details.)

Dosage and Administration

Dosage. Triflupromazine 25 mg is the therapeutic equivalent of 2 mg of haloperidol. Dosage should be titrated to the individual's need and tolerance. For the symptomatic management of psychosis, the usual initial IM dose is 60 mg given in divided doses. Dosage may be titrated upward to a maximum IM dose of 150 mg/day. In children the usual initial IM dose is 0.2 to 0.25 mg/kg/day and should not exceed 10 mg/day. The safety and efficacy of triflupromazine in children younger than 2 1/2 years old have not been established.

Nausea and Vomiting. The usual antiemetic dose at the initiation of treatment is 5 to 15 mg as a single dose. This may be repeated every 4 to 6 hours to a maximum daily dose of 60 mg/day. In the debilitated or elderly patient the initial dose is 2.5 mg IM with the maximum dose generally not exceeding 15 mg/day. The usual IV dosage of triflupromazine hydrochloride for the treatment of nausea and vomiting is 1 mg repeated up to a maximum of 3 mg/day. The dosage in children older than 2 1/2 years of age is 0.2 to 0.25 mg/kg/day given in divided doses. The maximum recommended dose as an antiemetic is 10 mg/day.

Administration. Triflupromazine hydrochloride is administered by IM or IV injection. IV administration of triflupromazine hydrochloride is not recommended for children.

Preparation

Triflupromazine hydrochloride (*Vesprin*)
  Parenteral, injection
    10 mg/mL, 20 mg/mL

PSYCHOSTIMULANTS 6

GENERAL STATEMENT

The psychostimulants (e.g., the amphetamines and methylphenidate) are sympathomimetic amines with significant central nervous system (CNS) stimulant activity. Their sympathomimetic activity includes increase in blood pressure, bronchodilation, mydriasis, contraction of the urinary bladder sphincter, and respiratory stimulation. The mechanism of action for the CNS effects of stimulants is not fully known. It is known, however, that in peripheral tissues the drug acts by a release of norepinephrine from stores in adrenergic nerve terminals and by directly stimulating α- and β-receptors sites.

In the CNS, the drugs appear to stimulate the cerebral cortex and reticular formation. In high doses, they cause the release of CNS dopamine and serotonin, in addition to the release of norepinephrine. It is known that in the brain, stimulants inhibit monoamine oxidase and it has been suggested that this may be responsible for the mood-elevating effects of these drugs. Owing to their CNS effects, the drugs produce mild euphoria, reduction of fatigue, increase in mental alertness, and an increase in motor activity. These effects may permit an increase in mental and physical activity. These stimulant effects are often followed by depression and fatigue. Psychostimulants produce a reduction in appetite, and chronic use may be associated with weight loss. Tolerance to all these effects occurs with repeated use. Thus, their use as weight reduction aids is quite limited.

DRUG INTERACTION

Fatalities and near fatalities have occurred in patients receiving stimulants and a monoamine oxidase inhibitor (MAOI: phenelzine, tranylcypromine, etc.) concurrently. An MAOI with intrinsic amphetamine-like activity such as tranylcypromine is likely to be more dangerous in this regard. Hypertensive crisis, hyperpyrexia, cerebral hemorrhage, and seizures have been reported with this combined therapy. Amphetamines can reverse the hypotensive effects of guanethidine, as has been demonstrated in a variety of animal models, and in small, open human studies.

Methylphenidate appears to inhibit the metabolism of tricyclic antidepressants and may increase their blood levels significantly. The anticoagulant action of ethyl biscoumacetate (dicumarol) may possibly be enhanced by methylphenidate. However, results from two controlled studies are conflicting. It has been proposed that methylphenidate inhibits the metabolism of phenytoin, but there is some question as to the significance of this interaction.

In patients ingesting large amounts of amphetamines, (e.g., amphetamine abusers) one should be alert for an enhanced pressor response to intravenous norepinephrine. There is a mutually inhibitory effect of amphetamines and phenothiazines (PTZs); amphetamines may inhibit the antipsychotic effect of PTZs, and PTZs may antagonize the anorectic effect and amphetamine-induced mood and locomotor symptoms. Case reports suggest that lithium carbonate appears to inhibit amphetamine "highs" and reverse weight reduction due to amphetamines. Urinary alkalinizers (e.g., sodium bicarbonate) may diminish urinary elimination of unionized amphetamine, resulting in relatively more of the drug being eliminated by hepatic metabolism, thus enhancing (or at least prolonging) amphetamine efficacy and toxicity. Acidification of the urine prevents amphetamine renal tubular reabsorption, thereby increasing amphetamine urinary elimination. Urinary acidification has been used therapeutically for amphetamine overdose.

Table 6–1 summarizes the established interactions between the psychostimulants and other drugs.

AMPHETAMINE

Pharmacokinetics

Amphetamine sulfate is readily absorbed from the gastrointestinal (GI) tract. It is widely distributed into most body tissues and fluids with high concentrations occurring in the cerebrospinal fluid (CSF) and brain. The effects last anywhere from 4 to 24 hours. Amphetamine is excreted in the urine.

Uses

Amphetamine is used in the treatment of depression, narcolepsy, and attention deficit disorder with hyperactivity in children.

Cautions

Adverse Effects. Paradoxical psychological reactions may include worsening of depression and increased agitation in depressed patients. Amphetamines may exacerbate psychosis, and in large doses or chronic use cause psychosis; therefore, they should be used cautiously or even avoided in individuals with psychotic symptoms. Adverse effects also include nausea, irritability, insomnia, nervousness, talkativeness, increased libido, increased motor activity, blurred vision, dizziness, headaches, and hyperexcitability. Changes in blood pressure and cardiac rhythm may also occur. In general, tolerance develops to amphetamines, but chronic use may be associated with congestive heart failure or ventricular hypertrophy, or both.

Precautions and Contraindications. The possibility of dependence should be considered prior to the administration of amphetamines. Furthermore, patients should be cautioned about engaging in hazardous activity such as driving a motor vehicle or operating machinery while under the influence of amphetamines. In fact, amphetamines may impair a patient's ability to perform such hazardous activity or other activities requiring mental alertness or physical coordination. Sustained administration or large doses of amphetamine may produce hallucinations, depression, fatigue, alterations in blood pressure, and disorientation. Seizures and coma in large doses may also occur. Likewise, abrupt discontinuation of amphetamine may produce psychomotor depression, lethargy, and psychosis.

In general, amphetamine is considered to be contraindicated in patients with a history of drug abuse, hypertension of moderate or severe degree, cardiovascular disease which is symptomatic (such as advanced arteriosclerosis), hyperthyroidism, or glaucoma. Prolonged administration of amphetamine to children has been associated with a retardation in growth and weight. Patients should be closely monitored for these effects.

Pregnancy, Fertility, and Lactation. In general, amphetamines should be avoided during pregnancy, in particular during the first trimester, as the drug readily crosses the placenta. With regular use, there is also the risk of the infant experiencing withdrawal symptoms during the first week of life.

Acute Toxicity

Death from amphetamine overdose usually results from cardiovascular collapse or from seizures. Overdosage usually includes such

Table 6–1.
Drug Interactions With CNS Stimulants (Amphetamines, Methylphenidate)

Combination	Interaction Effect	Mechanism/ Comment	Clinical Significance
Anticoagulants, oral (dicumarol) with methylphenidate	May ↑ anticoagulant effect (↑ prothrombin time)	Methylphenidate may inhibit metabolism of dicumarol Conflicting results from two controlled studies	?
Anticonvulsants (phenytoin, primidone) with methylphenidate	May ↑ serum phenytoin levels (?)	In vitro studies: methylphenidate may be competitive inhibitor of hepatic metabolism of phenytoin Clinical experience and studies suggest combination is usually safe	?
Guanethidine–amphetamines, methylphenidate	↓ Hypotensive effects of guanethidine	Mechanism controversial Arrhythmias also shown in case report Satisfactory blood pressure control cannot be obtained with this combination; shift to alternative antihypertensive agent or ↑ guanethidine dose	Yes
Lithium-amphetamines	May inhibit amphetamine"highs" and reverse weight reduction from amphetamines	Mechanism? Case report only	?
MAOIs–amphetamines, methylphenidate	Fatal reactions: hypertensive crisis, hyperpyrexia, cerebral hemorrhage, seizures, etc. (see also Chap 2)	Probably ↑ norepinephrine at synaptic cleft Avoid this combination	Yes

		Hypertensive reactioon may occur for up to several weeks after discontinuing MAOIs Phentolamine (Regitine) for treatment of servere hypertension Methylphenidate-MAOIs: reactions may be less severe	
Methyldopa with amphetamines, other sympathomimetic amines	↓ Antihypertensive effect of methylodopa Methyldopa may ↑ pressor effects of sympathomimetic amines	Amphetamines act indirectly by displacing norepinephrine to site of action It is better to avoid this combination	?
Norepinephrine (Levophed)-amphetamines	May enhance pressor response to IV norepinephrine	Mechanism ? This was shown with patients ingesting large amounts of amphetamines (the effect of chronic amphetamine use in normal "therapeutic" doses??)	?
Oral contraceptives–methylphenidate	May ↑ action of oral contraceptive, and side effects (e.g., fluid retention, diabetogenic action, hypertensive effect, risk of thromboembolic disorders)	↓ Hepatic metabolism of both the estrogen and progestogen components	?
Pempidine-amphetamines	Pempidine may ↑ sensitivity to amphetamines and sympathomimetic amines	Mechanism ? These agents should only be given concomitantly to antagonize hypotensive effects of pempidine.	?

(Continued.)

Table 6–1 (cont.).

Combination	Interaction Effect	Mechanism/ Comment	Clinical Significance
Phenothiazines, haloperidol–amphetamines	Amphetamines may ↓ antipsychotic effects of PTZ and haloperidol PTZ, etc. may antagonize pharmacologic effects of amphetamines	Mechanism ? Avoid combination	Yes
Tricyclic antidepressant (TCA)–methylphenidate	↑ Serum levels of TCA	Inhibition of TCA metabolism Combination may exhibit improvement in clinical symptoms of ↑ adverse effects	?
Urinary acidifiers (Ammonium chloriide, sodium acid phosphate) with amphetamines	↑ Elimination of amphetamines with concomitant ↓ in duration of action	↓ Urine pH prevents amphetamine renal tubular reabsorption Interaction has been exploited therapeutically for amphetamine overdose	Yes
Urinary alkalinizers (sodium bicarbonate, sodium acetate, potassium citrate) with amphetamines	Prolong effects of amphetamines	↓ Urinary elimination of unionized amphetamines Avoid agents which may alkalinize urine, particularly in overdose situations	? Yes

manifestations as flushing or pallor, tachypnea, fluctuations in pulse and blood pressure, tremor, palpitations, and cardiac arrhythmias such as extrasystoles, heart block, circulatory collapse, and chest pain. Hyperpyrexia is a frequent sign. There may be delirium, confusion, or acute psychotic manifestations such as delusions and hallucinations. Hallucinations may be visual or auditory. There may be anxiety and suicidal or homicidal ideation along with paranoid ideation. There may be changes in mood and loose associations. In most cases, the psychosis clears within approximately 1 week. Treatment of acute amphetamine overdosage is nonspecific and includes the administration of neuroleptics and minimization of environmental stimuli. In significant overdosage general supportive measures should be undertaken. Furthermore, the drug should be removed from the GI tract by lavage. Excretion may be hastened by acidification of the urine.

Chronic Toxicity

Tolerance develops with prolonged administration of the usual therapeutic levels. In addition, habituation and physical or psychic dependence may develop. The drug may be abused on account of its euphorigenic effects or for the general lessening of fatigue and CNS stimulation it provides. Symptoms of chronic abuse include changes in appetite, somnolence, emotional lability, social isolation, and deterioration in role or occupational functioning.

Dosage and Administration

Dosage. In general, the effective dosage varies widely among patients. The lowest possible dose should be used at the initiation of treatment. Dosage should be titrated to the individual's need and tolerance. In the treatment of narcolepsy, individual dosage may vary between 5 and 60 mg/day, depending on the patient's tolerance, age, and response. In general, this dosage is divided into two or three daily doses every 4 to 6 hours. The initial dosage in patients older than 12 years of age is 10 mg; this dose can be adjusted upward as tolerated and required. In patients 6 to 12 years of age the initial dose is 5 mg/day. Dosage is titrated upward at weekly intervals by 5 mg until an optimal response or side effects limit further dose increases. A dosage of 5 mg once or twice a day is used in the treatment of attention deficit disorder in children older than 12 years of age. This may be increased by 5-mg increments each week until an optimal response is obtained or until further increase is limited by side effects.

In children 3 to 5 years of age, the initial dosage is 2.5 mg/day with the daily dosage being increased by 2.5 mg at weekly intervals.

Administration. Amphetamines are administered orally. In general, they are given at least 6 hours before the initiation of sleep to avoid impairment of sleep.

Preparations

Amphetamine combinations
- Oral capsules
  - 6.25 mg with dextroamphetamine 6.25 mg (*Biphetamine*)
  - 10 mg with dextroamphetamine 10 mg (*Biphetamine 20*)

Amphetamine sulphate
- Oral tablets
  - 5 mg, 10 mg

DEXTROAMPHETAMINE

Uses

Dextroamphetamine is the dextrorotatory-isomer of amphetamine; it is three to four times more potent than the levorotatory isomer. Dextroamphetamine is used in the treatment of narcolepsy, in the treatment of attention deficit disorder with hyperactivity, and in the treatment of depression.

Dosage and Administration

Dosage. The effective dose varies from individual to individual and for this reason dosage should be titrated to response and tolerance. In the treatment of narcolepsy, the usual initial dose is 10 mg/day in patients 12 years of age and older; this is increased by 10-mg increments at weekly intervals. The ultimate dosage may range from 5 to 16 mg/day. In patients between the ages of 6 and 12 years, the initial dosage is 5 mg/day increased by weekly increments of 5 mg. In the treatment of attention deficit disorder, in children older than 6 years of age, the initial dosage is 5 mg once or twice a day increased by 5-mg increments until an optimal response is attained. In children between 3 and 5 years of age, the initial dose is 2.5 mg increased by 2.5 mg at weekly intervals until an optimal response is obtained.

Administration. Dextroamphetamine is administered orally.

Preparations

Dextroamphetamine combinations
  Oral capsules
    6.25 mg with amphetamine 6.25 mg (*Biphetamine 12½*)
    10 mg with amphetamine 10 mg (*Biphetamine 20*)
Dextroamphetamine sulfate
  Oral capsules, extended-release (*Dexedrine Spansule*)
    5 mg, 10 mg, 15 mg
  Elixir (*Dexedrine*)
    5 mg/5 mL
  Tablets
    5 mg (*Dexedrine, Ferndex, Oxydess*)
    10 mg, 15 mg (*dextroamphetamine sulfate tablets*)

METHYLPHENIDATE

Pharmacology

The actions of methylphenidate are similar to those of the amphetamines. Methylphenidate produces CNS and respiratory stimulation and has sympathomimetic activity.

Pharmacokinetics

Methylphenidate is well absorbed from the GI tract with clinical effects persisting for 3 to 6 hours after the administration of oral tablets. Effects last approximately 8 hours after the administration of extended-release tablets. Peak plasma levels are reached in 1 to 2 hours; ingestion with food may accelerate absorption. Methylphenidate is primarily metabolized by hydroxylation to ritalinic acid, followed by renal excretion.

Uses

Methylphenidate is used in the treatment of attention deficit disorder, narcolepsy, and depression.

Cautions

Adverse Effects. In general, adverse effects are dose-related. The most frequent side effects are nervousness and insomnia. These usually respond to dose reduction or by administering the bulk of the dose in the morning so that it is less likely to interfere with sleep. Other adverse effects include a reduction in appetite (over prolonged administration this may be associated with weight loss), nausea, palpitations, dizziness, headache, and restlessness. There may be cardiac arrhythmias with tachycardia and angina pectoris, and fluctuations in blood pressure and pulse. Prolonged administration to children with attention deficit disorder with hyperactivity may produce difficulty with weight gain and impaired growth.

Precautions and Contraindications. Tolerance and psychological dependence may develop in patients taking methylphenidate for prolonged periods of time. Furthermore, psychosis can develop with prolonged administration; this may include auditory and visual hallucinations. Methylphenidate may also exacerbate anxiety in patients with a preexisting history of anxiety symptoms or anxiety disorders. Patients with moderate or severe hypertension may experience exacerbation with the administration of methylphenidate. Methylphenidate may affect patients with preexisting seizure disorders and exacerbate the condition or produce electroencephalographic (EEG) abnormalities. Caution should be exercised in administering this drug to patients with a known history of drug abuse or dependence.

Acute Toxicity

Manifestations. Manifestations of methylphenidate overdose are similar to those seen in amphetamine overdose. Prominent signs and symptoms are cardiovascular symptoms such as hypertension, arrhythmias, palpitations, and flushing. There may be confusion, delirium, hallucinations, and euphoria. Other symptoms may include headache, vomiting, agitation, prominent sweating, fever, tremors, and hyperreflexia. Ultimately, there may be seizures which may be followed by coma. In treating methylphenidate overdosage, the stomach should be emptied of any possible remaining drug by gastric lavage. General physiologic support should be provided, including the maintenance of adequate respiration and circulation. The patient should be placed in an environment which minimizes stimulation and treated if necessary with neuroleptics.

Methylphenidate may inhibit the metabolism of certain drugs such as antidepressants, anticonvulsants, anticoagulants, and warfarin (Coumadin). Care should be exercised in patients receiving MAOIs. Methylphenidate may raise the serum concentrations of anticonvulsants and warfarin.

Dosage and Administration

Dosage. Doses of methylphenidate should be titrated to the individual's need and tolerance. The usual initial dosage is 5 mg twice a day increased by 5 to 10 mg at weekly intervals. Maximum dosage rarely exceeds 60 mg/day. In general, as with the amphetamines, the drug should be discontinued episodically to reassess continued benefit from ongoing drug treatment. Often drug therapy can be discontinued when a child reaches adolescence. In the treatment of narcolepsy, the usual adult dosage is 10 mg two to three times a day given 30 minutes before meals. Some patients may require up to 60 mg/day or as little as 10 mg/day.

Extended-release preparations should be initiated only after the patient has achieved stable daily dosing on standard preparations. The extended release tablets may be given at 8-hour intervals in the treatment of attention deficit disorder with hyperactivity in children 6 years of age and older.

Administration. Methylphenidate is administered orally.

Preparations

Methylphenidate hydrochloride
- Oral tablets (*Ritalin Hydrochloride*)
  - 5 mg, 10 mg, 20 mg
- Tablets, extended-release (*Ritalin-SR*)
  - 20 mg

MISCELLANEOUS AGENTS 7

Enzyme Inhibitor (Prolactin)

BROMOCRIPTINE MESYLATE

Chemistry

Bromocriptine mesylate is an ergot-derived dopamine receptor agonist and thus inhibits prolactin and growth hormone secretions.

Pharmacology

Bromocriptine activates dopaminergic receptors in the neostriatum of the central nervous system (CNS). This effect may be helpful in the treatment of parkinsonian syndrome, galactorrhea, neuroleptic malignant syndrome (NMS), and possibly tardive dyskinesia.

Pharmacokinetics

Absorption. Approximately 28% of the oral dose is absorbed from the gastrointestinal (GI) tract after oral administration. However, there is substantial first pass metabolism resulting in only 6% of the orally administered doses reaching the systemic circulation. Peak concentration and effect is reached in 1 to 2 hours.

Distribution. Bromocriptine is 90% to 95% bound to serum albumin. The elimination half-life is biphasic: the initial phase is 3.0 to 4.5 hours with 45 to 50 hours for the terminal phase. Bromocriptine is completely metabolized in the liver. New metabolites are not pharmacologically active or toxic. Bromocriptine and its metabolites are excreted principally in the feces via biliary elimination. Within approximately 5 days, 85% of the dose is excreted.

Uses

Parkinsonian syndrome. Bromocriptine, like other dopaminergic drugs, is useful in the treatment of Parkinson's disease or parkinsonian-like symptoms produced by the extrapyramidal effects of neuroleptics. Because of the significant risk of adverse side effects, bromocriptine is rarely used as the primary treatment; however, it can be useful as an adjunct in treatment-resistant cases, or when trying to lower the dose of the primary drug (e.g., an anticholinergic).

Neuroleptic Malignant Syndrome. This rare syndrome is associated with the use of neuroleptic drugs, and is characterized by hyperthermia, delirium or stupor, autonomic instability, and muscular symptoms. The last include rigidity, catatonia, tremor, dysarthria, elevated serum creatine phosphokinase, and sometimes myoglobinuria. This syndrome may have a mortality rate as high as 20%. Treatment consists of immediate discontinuation of any neuroleptic drug, physiologic monitoring, and supportive care in an intensive care unit (ICU) setting. Recommended drug treatment includes intravenous (IV) dantrolene and oral bromocriptine. These drugs are often used in combination in this setting. Occasionally, amantadine is used if the patient has not responded well to the above treatment.

Galactorrhea. Owing to bromocriptine's inhibitory effect on prolactin secretion, it is useful in the short term for inhibiting galactorrhea.

Tardive Dyskinesia. This syndrome of involuntary movements is associated with long-term use of neuroleptic drugs (see Chapter 4). No drug treatment has proved satisfactory, but, bromocriptine appears to improve symptoms in 20% of patients. The mechanism of action is thought to be an inhibition of dopamine synthesis and release secondary to its action on dopamine presynaptic autoreceptors.

Cautions

Adverse Effects. Adverse effects are common, dose-related, and more frequent when dosage exceeds 20 mg/day. They are usually moderate in severity and can be minimized by using the lowest possible dose, and also by initiating treatment at a low dose and titrating upward.

GI Effects. Dry mouth, metallic taste, nausea, vomiting, anorexia, abdominal discomfort, indigestion, constipation, or diarrhea may all occur. Dysphagia also has been reported.

Nervous System Effects. Adverse effects have included headaches, drowsiness, fatigue, insomnia, faintness, lightheadedness, and sedation. Confusion, hallucinations, and delusions may occur at higher doses. Mania has also been reported as has depression with severe suicidal thoughts.

Cardiovascular Effects. Hypotension commonly accompanies bromocriptine treatment. The drug may produce syncope, postural hypotension, shock, or exacerbation of angina. Palpitations and arrhythmias with tachycardia or bradycardia have been reported.

Other Adverse Effects. Livido reticularis is more common with bromocriptine than with levodopa. Bromocriptine may induce burning discomfort of the eyes, diplopia, rash, and urticaria. Bromocriptine may also cause transient increases in serum concentrations of aspartate aminotransferase (AST, SGOT), alaine aminotransferase (ALT, SGPT), γ-glutamyltransferase (GGT), creatine kinase (CK), alkaline phosphatase, uric acid, and blood urea nitrogen (BUN).

Precautions and Contraindications

Blood pressure should be monitored periodically, in particular after initiation of treatment or recent increases in dosage. Care should be exercised in those patients receiving other hypotensive drugs. Patients should be warned that bromocriptine may impair their ability to perform activities that require mental alertness or physical coordination such as operating machinery or driving a motor vehicle.

Hepatic, cardiovascular, renal function, and hematopoietic function should be monitored prior to the initiation of therapy and periodically thereafter.

Bromocriptine should be used with caution in patients with impaired liver or renal function since its safety has not been established in these patients. Some preparations of bromocriptine mesylate contain sodium bisulfite, a sulfite that may cause allergic reactions including anaphylaxis and life-threatening or severe asthmatic episodes in susceptible individuals. While the overall prevalence of this is low, it is higher in patients with asthma.

Drug Interactions

Preliminary clinical evidence indicates that the combined use of bromocriptine and alcohol may enhance the likelihood of GI side effects or alcohol intolerance. Patients should be warned to abstain from alcohol, because of the severe side effects. Griseofulvin may increase the metabolism of bromocriptine, thus reducing the drug activity. Anecdotal experience implies that the phenothiazines may inhibit the effectiveness of bromocriptine for treatment of certain prolactin-secreting tumors. If possible, avoid the combination.

Acute Toxicity

Overdosage of bromocriptine may cause nausea, vomiting, and severe hypotension. Treatment of overdosage consists of emptying the stomach by aspiration and lavage and administration of IV fluids to treat hypotension.

Dosage and Administration

Dosage

Parkinsonian syndrome. Therapy is initiated at a low dosage and titrated upward until a therapeutic response is achieved. The usual initial dosage is 1.25 mg twice a day. The safety of bromocriptine in dosages greater than 100 mg/day has not been established.

Neuroleptic Malignant Syndrome. Bromocriptine 2.5 to 5.0 mg has been given 2 to 6 times per day.

Galactorrhea. Bromocriptine 1.25 mg twice a day is usually used.

Tardive Dyskinesia. Bromocriptine 0.75 to 7.5 mg/day is used. Doses as high as 20 mg/day have been used.

Administration. Bromocriptine mesylate is administered orally with food.

Preparations

Bromocriptine mesylate (*Parlodel*)
- Oral capsules
  - 5 mg
- Tablets
  - 2.5 mg

Anxiolytic

BUSPIRONE HYDROCHLORIDE

Buspirone is a novel anxiolytic which differs structurally and pharmacologically from the benzodiazepines.

Pharmacology

Nervous System Effects. Buspirone is an anxiolytic agent without anticonvulsant or muscle relaxant capabilities. Furthermore, it does not produce significant sedation or impairment in psychomotor function. Its mechanism of action is unknown. It appears, however, to affect a variety of sites in the CNS and to affect a variety of neurotransmitters including the dopaminergic, cholinergic, serotonergic, and α-adrenergic systems. It does not appear to be a benzodiazepine receptor ligand. Furthermore, it does not appear to modulate affinity to the benzodiazepine receptor or to modulate γ-aminobutyric acid (GABA) binding. Buspirone does have high affinity for serotonin type 1 receptors and moderate affinity for dopamine type 2 receptors.

Buspirone has high affinity for the serotonin type 1A receptor and acts as a partial agonist or a mixed agonist-antagonist. This action appears to be involved in the inhibition of the dorsal raphe, an effect also produced by benzodiazepines (via a different mechanism); this may be the mechanism for anxiolysis. Buspirone also has mixed dopamine agonist and antagonist activity; however, the contribution of this activity to anxiolytic effects is unknown.

Neuroendocrine Effects. Buspirone causes an increase in prolactin secretion; however, this is usually not clinically significant. Likewise, increases in somatotropin which are not usually clinically significant may occur.

Cardiovascular Effects. Tachycardia or palpitations may occur in a small number of patients taking buspirone; however, generally, there are no important electrocardiographic (ECG) changes or other changes in vital signs.

Pharmacokinetics

Absorption. Following oral administration, buspirone is rapidly and almost completely absorbed from the GI tract. After absorption there is extensive metabolism by the liver with approximately 4% of an administered dose reaching the circulation in an unchanged form. The amount of unchanged available drug may be increased when the drug is administered with food, though this delays absorption.

Distribution. Distribution of buspirone is widespread in tissue and fluid, with large concentrations of buspirone and

1-pyrimidinylpiperazine, the active metabolite of buspirone, found in the brain. Buspirone is 95% bound to plasma proteins and is distributed in breast milk.

Elimination. The elimination half-life of buspirone ranges from 2 to 4 hours on average and is not significantly affected by the administration of the drug with food. The elimination half-life is increased in patients with hepatic or renal impairment. Buspirone is metabolized in the liver via oxidation and subsequently via conjugation. After metabolism the drug is excreted principally in the urine with some metabolites also being found in the feces; however, dosage reduction may not be necessary in patients with mild to moderate renal impairment.

Uses

Anxiety Disorders. Buspirone is effective in the treatment of anxiety disorders, in particular generalized anxiety disorder where symptoms have been present continously for at least 1 month. Its efficacy is best established in short-term use of 3 to 4 weeks' duration, but, many patients have been treated for periods in excess of 1 year without significant loss of clinical efficacy. In all cases of prolonged drug treatment, continuous reassessment of the need for the medication should be performed. In patients with generalized anxiety disorder, buspirone is as effective as conventionally used doses of benzodiapines and more effective than placebo in reducing anxiety symptoms. Buspirone is associated with less severe sedation and psychomotor impairment than is found with the benzodiazepines. It has little liability for dependence and little interaction with alcohol. It appears to have none of the abuse potential associated with benzodiazepines. Furthermore, buspirone appears to diminish anger and hostility in some patients when it occurs as part of their generalized anxiety disorder. It reduces these symptoms without producing disinhibition. Buspirone has a slower onset of therapeutic action than is associated with benzodiazepines. The onset of the therapeutic effect is usually gradual over 1 to 4 weeks; for this reason some patients may need initial brief management of their anxiety with benzodiazepines. Furthermore, some patients treated with buspirone may need adjunctive, short-term benzodiazepines for sleep induction since buspirone is not an effective hypnotic.

Buspirone has not been shown to be effective for panic disorder. The effectiveness for generalized anxiety disorder may be reduced in patients who have been previously treated with benzodiazepines. Recent studies suggest that buspirone may also be effective in treating major depression.

Cautions

In general, buspirone is well tolerated. Headache, drowsiness, lightheadedness, tinnitus, and dizziness are the most common adverse effects of buspirone. Also common, and seen in 10% of patients are insomnia, nervousness, drowsiness, and fatigue, along with GI effects such as nausea. The elderly may be more likely to develop such side effects, though, generally, elderly patients tolerate buspirone well. The incidence of adverse reactions is more frequent with higher dosages, but, with time most side effects appear to diminish.

Nervous System Effects. Other nervous system side effects include excitement, depression, impaired concentration, nightmares, weakness, confusion, anger, hostility, impaired coordination, tremor, numbness, and paresthesias. Insomnia and nervousness are particularly problematic when total daily dosage exceeds 100 mg and sedation may become more problematic as dosages exceed 20 mg/day. These, however, are mostly likely to occur during the time of drug initiation or dose increase and tend to remit with time.

GI Effects. Nausea is the most common GI side effect. Less frequent effects include dry mouth, diarrhea, constipation, vomiting; even less frequent are reduction in appetite, flatulence, salivation, and, rarely, irritable colon or rectal bleeding.

Cardiovascular Effects. Tachycardia, palpitations, and nonspecific chest pain have been reported.

Dermatologic Effects. Occasional reactions include pruritus, flushing, edema, easy bruising, rash, hair loss, facial edema, dry skin, and blisters.

Other Adverse Effects. Endocrine irregularities such as amenorrhea, menstrual spotting, galactorrhea, and thyroid abnormalities have occasionally occurred in patients. There may also be changes in libido, and in urinary function, including frequency, hesitancy, or dysuria; furthermore, there may be arthralgias, hyperventilation, and dyspnea. There may be elevations in serum aminotransferases (AST, ALT). Blurred vision may occur in some patients receiving buspirone.

Precautions and Contraindications. Buspirone may impair the ability to operate machinery or drive a motor vehicle or perform other activities that require either mental alertness or physical coordination. Patients should be cautioned to avoid such activities if they experience these effects from buspirone. In general, these effects are less common with buspirone than with other anxiolytics. Likewise, interactions with alcohol are less frequent than with other anxiolytics; however, patients should be cautioned about engaging in hazardous activities while under the influence of buspirone and alcohol. Buspirone should not be administered to patients currently receiving a monoamine oxidase inhibitor (MAOI). Because buspirone does not have cross-tolerance with benzodiazepines, it cannot be used to prevent withdrawal symptoms in patients who have been maintained on these other anxiolytics.

Mutagenicity and Carcinogenicity. No evidence of mutagenesis or carcinogenesis has been reported with buspirone.

Pregnancy, Fertility, and Lactation. There is no evidence that buspirone causes impaired fertility or fetal abnormality in animals. The drug and its active metabolites are excreted into breast milk in animals. Concentrations in human breast milk are unknown. Buspirone should be used with caution in nursing women and should be used only when the benefits clearly exceed the risks in pregnant women. Buspirone is classified in the Food and Drug Administration (FDA) pregnancy category B.

Chronic Toxicity

There appears to be little physical or psychological dependence with long-term administration of buspirone. Furthermore, there is little development of tolerance. Patients maintained on the drug for 6 to 12 weeks do not have a withdrawal syndrome following sudden discontinuation of buspirone. Despite these observations, patients with a history of prior drug abuse or dependence should be carefully evaluated during buspirone therapy for signs of dependence, escalation of drug usage, drug-seeking behavior, or the development of tolerance. Furthermore, the possibility of withdrawal developing after the abrupt discontinuation of high doses of buspirone should be considered.

Acute Toxicity

The lethal dose of buspirone for humans is unknown. Overdose may produce nausea, vomiting, drowsiness, miosis, dizziness, and gastric distention. Treatment involves symptomatic and supportive care with the stomach being emptied by gastric lavage.

Drug Interactions

Concurrent administration of MAOIs and buspirone is not recommended. Two weeks should elapse following the discontinuation of an MAOI and the administration of buspirone, to prevent hypertensive reactions which have been found to develop when both drugs are administered together. Fluoxetine is a selective inhibitor of serotonin neuronal uptake and may block the serotonergic activity of busiprone, thus decreasing the pharmacologic effects of buspirone. Coadministration of trazodone with buspirone may result in a significant elevation in serum ALT in some patients. This does not contraindicate the coadministration of these two drugs, but, there should be a careful monitoring of liver function tests. Coadministration of haloperidol with buspirone may produce elevated blood levels of haloperidol. Food may delay absorption of buspirone and decrease first-pass metabolism in the liver. The clinical significance of this is unknown but it does not appear to produce a significant increase in toxicity or other adverse effects. Buspirone does not alter blood alcohol concentration or potentiate alcohol-induced impairment. Likewise, buspirone appears to have minimal interaction with benzodiazepines. However, despite the absence of data suggesting an interaction between benzodiazepines and buspirone, the effects of the combination of these two drug groups have not been fully evaluated; until this is forthcoming, caution should be exercised in patients receiving buspirone and benzodiazepines. Care should also be exercised when buspirone and other CNS depressants are coadministered, because while no significant interaction between buspirone and other CNS depressants (such as antihistamines, sedative-hypnotics, or analgesics) have been documented, these also have not been fully evaluated.

Dosage and Administration

Dosage. The usual initial adult dosage for the treatment of anxiety disorders is 5 mg three times a day. Dosage may be increased by 5 to 10 mg every 3 to 4 days as tolerated and required. The manufacturer recommends that the dosage not exceed 60 mg/day. Optimal therapeutic relief of anxiety usually requires 3 to 4 weeks of drug therapy and may require up to 6 weeks. Early signs of symptomatic improvement may, however, occur as early as 1 to 2 weeks. Buspirone should be used with caution in patients with significant renal or hepatic impairment. Accumulation of active metabolites may occur in patients with moderate to severe renal impairment and may require adjustment of dosage.

Administration. Buspirone is administered orally.

Preparations

Buspirone hydrochloride (*Buspar*)
  Oral tablets
    5 mg, 10 mg

β-BLOCKERS

β-Blockers are used in psychiatry primarily for the treatment of akathisia and lithium-induced tremors. They are used in the treatment of specific anxiety disorders, such as social phobias and performance anxiety. β-Blockers may also have value in the treatment of hypertension due to cocaine overdose.

PROPRANOLOL

Propranolol is a nonselective β-adrenergic blocking agent which inhibits response to adrenergic stimuli via competitive blocking of β-adrenergic receptors. Propranolol has significant effects on the myocardium, reduces heart rate, and prevents exercise-induced increases in heart rate. Furthermore, propranolol decreases cardiac output and myocardial contractility, and increases cardiac volume and systolic ejection time. Long-term administration produces a reduction in peripheral resistance. These cardiovascular effects must be kept in mind when propranolol is administered for the control of either akathesia or lithium-induced tremor.

Pharmacokinetics

Absorption. While propranolol is almost completely absorbed from the GI tract, there are wide variations in plasma concentrations among individuals. The extended-release preparations have a slower rate of absorption and greater hepatic metabolism which results in lower serum concentrations. The slow-release preparations produce constant blood levels for approximately 12 hours.

Distribution. Propranolol is widely distributed throughout the body and readily crosses the blood-brain barrier. More than 90% of propranolol is bound to plasma proteins.

Elimination. The elimination half-life varies widely. Propranolol is metabolized in the liver and excreted in the bile.

Uses

The psychiatric uses of propranolol include the treatment of anxiety, lithium-induced tremor, and akathisia. Propranolol is also useful as an antagonist to the sympathomimetic effects of cocaine toxicity. For anxiety, propranolol appears to be useful in those patients with somatic symptoms of anxiety. The blocking of tremor, palpitations, and tachycardia may alter the patient's perception of his or her own mental state and may succeed in reducing anxiety. This appears to be most successful in patients with social phobias or performance anxieties, rather than in general anxiety disorder. Propranolol is also used in the treatment of hypertension, angina, and cardiac arrhythmias such as supraventricular arrhythmias, and ventricular tachycardias. It is also used in the treatment of hypertrophic subaortic stenosis and pheochromocytoma. Propranolol is also used in short-term treatment of arrhythmias and tachycardia associated with thyrotoxicosis. Myocardial infarction patients are also treated with long-term administration of propranolol to minimize mortality. Propranolol is effective in the prophylaxis of common migraine headache. It is not, however, effective for migraine headaches once they have begun. Propranolol is also used in the treatment of essential tremor. It effectively reduces the amplitude of the tremor, but it is rare that complete tremor suppression occurs.

Cautions

Adverse Reactions. Adverse reactions usually occur soon after the initiation of therapy. They are more frequent and severe after IV administration.

Cardiovascular Effects. Bradycardia is the most common adverse cardiovascular effect. It may be accompanied by syncope, hypotension, shock, or angina. Congestive heart failure may be precipitated in patients with inadequate cardiac function. Abrupt discontinuation of propranolol may exacerbate angina.

Nervous System Effects. Long-term treatment with high doses of propranolol may produce lightheadedness, ataxia, dizziness, hearing loss, hypnagogic hallucinations, sleepiness, irritability, confusion, insomnia, mental depression, fatigue, and weakness.

GI Effects. Epigastric distress, nausea, vomiting, and diarrhea may occur in patients on long-term propranolol.

Hematologic Effects. Propranolol may produce a transient eosinophilia.

Other Adverse Effects. Propranolol may elevate serum BUN, lactic dehydrogenase (LDH), alkaline phosphatase, serum aminotransferases, and serum creatinine.

Precautions and Contraindications. Propranolol should be used with caution in patients with compromised cardiac function. Congestive heart failure may be precipitated by propranolol. Abrupt discontinuation of propranolol may induce or exacerbate angina and may precipitate myocardial infarction in patients with coronary artery disease. Propranolol may mask the signs of thyrotoxicosis. Propranolol should be used with caution in diabetics because it may block the signs and symptoms of hypoglycemia and may inhibit the insulin-releasing mechanism of the pancreas. Propranolol should also not be used in patients with bronchospastic disease because of its ability to inhibit bronchodilation. Propranolol may produce increased airway resistance and bronchospasm.

Pregnancy, Fertility, and Lactation. Low birth weights have been found in infants born to mothers who received propranolol throughout their pregnancy. There have also been infants with respiratory distress and hypoglycemia. Propranolol should only be prescribed during pregnancy when the benefits clearly exceed the risks. Propranolol is excreted into breast milk and may produce symptoms in a newborn.

Acute Toxicity

Manifestations. The principle manifestations of propranolol overdosage are bradycardia and severe hypotension. There may be a loss of consciousness and ultimately seizures, along with cardiac failure and bronchospasm.

Treatment. In general, treatment is supportive and symptomatic. The stomach should be emptied by gastric lavage. IV atropine may be given for symptomatic bradycardia. If this is inadequate, IV isoproterenol may be administered. Vasopressors, such as norepinephrine or dopamine, may be given for severe hypotension.

Drug Interactions

Agents that increase the effects of propranolol or atenolol, e.g., cimetidine and hydralazine, appear to reduce the hepatic first-pass extraction, decrease liver blood flow, and may inhibit hepatic metabolism of propranolol, leading to increased propranolol bioavailability. The oxidative metabolism of β-blockers may be inhibited by quinidine. Orthostatic hypotension has occurred during concurrent propranolol or atenolol therapy. With the phenothiazines (PTZs) there may be additive hypotensive activity. There also may be an increase in plasma concentrations of propranolol because of a reduction in serum clearance. The hypotensive effects of propranolol may be exaggerated with the coadministration of other antihypertensive agents such as diuretics.

Agents that decrease the effects of propranolol or atenolol, e.g., nonsteroidal anti-inflammatory drugs (NSAIDs) and salicylates, may reduce the antihypertensive action of β-blockers (propranolol, atenolol, and pindolol) due to possible inhibition of renal prostaglandin synthesis. Drugs such as phenobarbital, phenytoin, and rifampin, as well as smoking, induce hepatic biotransformation enzymes and may decrease plasma levels of β-blockers that are metabolized extensively (e.g., propranolol). Effects of β-blockers can be reversed by sympathomimetic drugs such as isoproterenol, norepinephrine, or dopamine. IV epinephrine use in patients on propranolol can result in a rapid blood pressure increase, as well as a significant fall in heart rate. Propranolol may also block the β-adrenergic stimulating effects of sympathomimetic agents. Aluminum salts, cholestyramine, and colestipol may decrease the absorption of β-blockers. Thyroid hormones may reduce the pharmacologic effects of propranolol. When converting a patient from a hypothyroid to a euthyroid state, the propranolol dosage may need to be increased. When a patient is being converted from a hyperthyroid to a euthyroid state, the propranolol dosage may need to be decreased.

Propranolol and atenolol increase the effects of the following agents: Insulin's hypoglycemic effects may be prolonged by noncardioselective β-blockers (e.g., propranolol, not atenolol). Propranolol and atenolol may increase the effect of lidocaine.

Elevated plasma levels with toxicity characterized by confusion, lethargy, and other CNS and cardiovascular symptoms may manifest.

Miscellaneous Drug Interactions

β-Blockers (e.g., propranolol, atenolol, etc.) and calcium channel blockers have additive effects on the cardiac conduction system. Combination therapy in patients with atrioventricular (AV) conduction abnormalities or with depressed left ventricular function should be avoided. Catecholamine-depleting drugs such as reserpine may have an additive effect with β-blockers. Excessive sympathetic blockade with vertigo, syncope, or postural hypotension may result. β-blockers seem to enhance the rebound hypertensive reaction following clonidine withdrawal. Also, this combination has uncommonly caused paradoxical hypertension.

Pharmacologic effects of both drugs may be increased during concurrent atenolol and disopyramide therapy. Haloperidol and propranolol coadministration has resulted in a severe hypotensive reaction. Propranolol may potentiate, counteract, or have no effect on the actions of nondepolarizing muscle relaxants. Chlorpromazine (CPZ) and thioridazine may inhibit the first-pass hepatic metabolism of propranolol and increase its pharmacologic effects; however, CPZ and thioridazine levels have also increased. Coadministration of propranolol and prazosin may increase the "first dose response" (acute postural hypotension) produced by prazosin. Nonselective β-blockers antagonize the bronchodilating effect of theophylline, and may reduce theophylline elimination. A clinical study showed that food enhances the bioavailability of propranolol as indicated by increased peak serum concentration. Interactions between β-blockers and other commonly used medications are shown in Table 7–1.

Dosage and Administration

Dosage. Dosage should be titrated to the individual's need and tolerance. The usual dosage for akathisia or tremor is 20 mg, two to three times a day. The response is variable with some patients requiring dosages ranging from 120 to 320 mg/day administered in three or more divided doses. Standard dosages have not been established for the treatment of anxiety disorders. For social phobias 20 to 40 mg, two to three times a day, is recommended. For performance or test anxiety, 10 to 20 mg as a single dose, taken 1 hour before the performance (or test), may be effective.

Table 7–1.
Drug Interactions With β-Blockers (Propranolol, Atenolol)

Combination	Interaction	Mechanism/ Comment	Clinical Significance
Aluminum salts with atenolol, propranolol, metoprolol	↓ Absorption of β-blockers (?)	Certain aluminum salts may decrease rate of gastric emptying	?
Amiodarone with metoprolol, propranolol (?)	↑ Pharmacologic effects of metoprolol, propranolol (?), etc	Mechanism unknown; possibly decreased hepatic metabolism and diminished first-pass effect	?
Ampicillin (ampicillin-like?) with atenolol	↓ Atenolol plasma concentration and pharmacologic effects	Mechanism unknown	?
Anesthetics, local–propranolol	↑ Incidence of adverse effects (e.g., tachycardia arrhythmias, angina), if long-term propranolol therapy was discontinued	Chronic β-blocker therapy should not be discontinued prior to use of local anesthetics (e.g., tetracaine, bupivacaine) Epinephrine — containing local anesthetics + nonselective β-blockers (e.g., propranolol) may cause severe hypertensive reactions	Yes
Anticholinergics, e.g., propantheline (Pro-Banthine)	May ↑ bioavailability of atenolol	Probably by slowing gut motility Anticholinergics may attenuate propranolol-induced bradycardia	?

		Animal study: propranolol may enhance likelihood of atropine delirium	
Anticoagulants, oral, e.g., warfarin (Coumadin)	May ↑ anticoagulant effect of warfarin	Mechanism unknown No clinical interventions appear required at this time	?
Antidiabetic agents (insulin) with nonselective β-blocker (e.g., propranolol)	Prolonged hypoglycemia with masking of hypoglycemic symptoms (i.e., tachycardi), but hypoglycemic sweating does not appear to be affected (or may even be increased) Induce hypertension during hypoglycemia Inhibition of insulin secretion (under certain conditions, e.g., insulinoma) Propranolol may ↑ impairment of peripheral circulation that diabetics may already have	Inhibition of hyperglycemic and cardiac stimulatory effects of epinephrine Blockade of the β^2-adrenergic (vasodilator) effects of epinephrine released in response to hypoglycemia leaving unopposed α-adrenergic (vasoconstrictor) effect (↑ blood pressure) Inhibition of β^2-receptor in pancreas Cardioselective β-blockers have less inhibitory effect on insulin secretion (e.g., atenolol, metoprolol) Long-term propranolol therapy (especially with thiazides) may reduce glucose tolerance (propranolol > metoprolol)	Yes

(Continued.)

Table 7–1. (cont.).

Combination	Interaction	Mechanism/ Comment	Clinical Significance
		Cardioselective agents are preferable in diabetic patients, but, they may exhibit nonselective β-blockade (if large doses are used) Phenformin may have a similar interaction with propranolol	
Antipyrine	↑ Antipyrine half-life	Propranolol reduces hepatic clearance of antipyrine (?)	?
Antithyroid drugs or radioiodine with propranolol	Plasma propranolol steady-state concentration increased significantly after correction of thyroid disorder (in hyperthyroid patients by antithyroid drugs, radioiodine, or surgery)	Adjust propranolol dosage in thyroid disorders during and after treatment	Yes
Barbiturates (e.g., pentobarbital, phenobarbital	↓ Bioavailability of propranolol (β-blockers metabolized by liver)	Barbiturate enhances enzyme induction and hepatic first-pass extraction If an interaction is suspected, consider a higher dose of β-blocker	Yes

Benzodiazepines (BZDs) (e.g., clorazepate, diazepam	Effects of certain BZDs may be increased by lipophilic lipophilic β-blockers (e.g., propranolol, metoprolol)	Inhibition of BZD hepatic metabolism by β-blockers has been proposed Use a β-blocker that does not interfere with BZD hepatic metabolism (e.g., atenolol)	?
Caffeine-propranolol	↑ Coffee-induced fall in heart rate	Mechanism? No special precautions appear necessary	?
Calcium salts, oral–atenolol	May alter pharmacokinetic parameters and ↓ pharmacologic effects of atenolol	Impaired GI absorption of atenolol, and possibly increase in area of distribution volume Long-term interaction effects clinically insignificant	
Carbamazepine (CBZ) (Tegretol)	↓ Pharmacologic effects of propranolol (?)	CBZ tends to increase serum levels of α^1-acid glycoprotein (which propranolol is bound with) CBZ may increase hepatic metabolism of β-blockers (theoretical consideration, clinical implication ??)	?

(Continued.)

Table 7–1 (cont.).

Combination	Interaction	Mechanism/ Comment	Clinical Significance
Cholestyramine, colestipol–propranolol	↓ Therapeutic and pharmacologic actions of propranolol	Possibly reduced GI absorption due to binding of propranolol to nonabsorbable anionic exchange resins Tailor propranolol dosage upward if needed, or stagger administration time	?
Cimetidine (Tagamet)-propranolol	↑ Plasma levels of propranolol and may ↑ pharmacodynamic effects	Cimetidine may reduce hepatic first-pass extraction and inhibit hepatic metabolism of propranolol Other β-blockers excreted extensively by kidneys (e.g., atenolol, nadolol) would not be much affected by cimetidine Ranitidine may be preferable to cimetidine in this case Antacids or sucralfate may also be suitable alternatives to cimetidine (separating their doses from β-blockers)	Yes

Clonidine (Catapres)–propranolol, atenolol	May enhance rebound hypertension following clonidine withdrawal Paradoxical hypertension Attenuation or addition of antihypertensive effect (?)	β-adrenergic (vasodilating) response of epinephrine blocked, resulting in exaggerated α-adrenergic (vasoconstrictor) response Labetalol (α-, β-blocking agent) may be useful in prevention of rebound hypertension following clonidine withdrawal Discontinue either agent gradually; preferably, discontinue clonidine first Closely monitor blood pressure after initiation or discontinuation of either drug	Yes
Diltiazem–propranolol, metoprolol	↑ Pharmacologic effects of propranolol, etc	Inhibition of oxidative metabolism by diltiazem (?)	?
Digitalis-propranolol	↑ Digitalis-induced bradycardia	? ↑ Sensitivity to action of propranolol Combination may be beneficial in some patients with AV reentrant tachycardia or in patients with angina who have abnormal ventricular function or enlarged hearts	?

(Continued.)

Table 7–1 (cont.).

Combination	Interaction	Mechanism/ Comment	Clinical Significance
Disopyramide-atenolol	Sinus bradycardia, hypotension, and pronounced decrease in cardiac output	Mechanism unknown (both agents may depress cardiac output) Atenolol may decrease clearance of disopyramide Interaction: controversial results	?
Dopamine-propranolol	Inhibits dopamine-induced increase in pulse rate	Blocks β-stimulatory effect of dopamine on heart	?
Epinephrine (Adrenalin) with nonselective β-blockers (e.g., propranolol)	Initial hypertensive episode, then bradycardia	With blockade of β-adrenergic effects of epinephrine using propranolol, α-adrenergic effects predominate Discontinue propranolol 3 days prior to epinephrine administration or avoid combination Cardioselective β-blockers have minimal effects on pressor response to epinephrine Treatment: Acutely monitor patient's vital signs Volume replacement	Yes

		IV chlorpromazine 1–5 mg; IV hydralazine; IV aminophylline 1 mg/kg; atropine	
Ergot alkaloids (e.g., dihydroergotamine [DHE-45], ergotamine, methysergide [Sansert] with propranolol	Peripheral ischemia (e.g., cold extremities, purple and painful feet) Paradoxical exacerbating headache	Propranolol blocks vasodilation pathway (peripheral β_2) Combination had been used in many cases with no problems; however, caution is warranted	Yes
Ethanol-propranolol	↑ CNS inhibition by ethanol Ethanol ↑ both elimination rate and bioavailability	Mechanism unknown; ethanol ↓ GI motility, or ↑ hepatic blood flow? Precautions appear unnecessary	?
Furosemide (Lasix)-propranolol	↑ Plasma levels and pharmacologic effects of propranolol	Mechanism unknown Atenolol does not appear to be affected by concurrent furosemide treatment	?
Glucagon	Propranolol partially inhibits hyperglycemic effect of glucagon Glucagon may be of value in treatment of excessive myocardial effects of propranolol	Mechanism unknown; probably propranolol inhibits hyperglycemic response to catecholamines and propranolol-induced decrease in hepatic gluconeogenesis β-Agonist effects of glucagon	?

(Continued.)

Table 7–1 (cont.).

Combination	Interaction	Mechanism/ Comment	Clinical Significance
Halofenate-propranolol	Decrease in steady-state plasma propranolol levels and its therapeutic actions	Mechanism: unknown Avoid adding halofenate to a patient stabilized on propranolol therapy for angina, otherwise, propranolol-withdrawal rebound phenomenon may occur	?
Haloperidol-propranolol	(See Table 4–1)		
Hydralazine-propranolol	May ↑ propranolol response (↑ bioavailability) (on fasting state)	Hydralazine may reduce first-pass metabolism of propranolol β-Blockers with low hepatic clearance or no first-pass metabolism (e.g., atenolol) appear not to exhibit this interaction	?
Isoniazid (Nydrazid)-propranolol	May ↑ pharmacologic effects of isoniazid	Mechanism ? Evidence comes from 1 healthy subject, control study	?

Isoproterenol (Isuprel)-propranolol	↓ Actions of isoproterenol	Mutually antagonistic effects Bronchodilation from isoproterenol is less likely to be reduced by cardioselective β-blockers (e.g., metoprolol)	Yes
Levodopa-propranolol	Propranolol may antagonize both hypotensive and positive inotropic effects of levodopa	Antagonizes β-adrenergic properties of dopamine	?
	May ↓↓ parkinsonian tremor	Propranolol may enhance (therapeutic) effect of levodopa (membrane-stabilizing properties?)	Yes
	May ↑↑ levodopa-induced growth hormone (GH) secretion	Patients on long-term combined therapy should be monitored with plasma GH assays	?
Lidocaine (lignocaine)-propranolol	↓↓ Lignocaine elimination (↑ its effects and toxicity, e.g., lethargy, confusion and other CNS, cardiovascular symptomatology, etc)	Mechanism? Case reports and studies in normal subjects have confirmed interaction Use combination with caution	Yes
Maprotiline (Ludiomil)-propranolol	May ↑ adverse effects of maprotiline, e.g., sedation, dry mouth,	Mechanism ? Reduce maprotiline dosage if needed	?

(Continued.)

Table 7–1 (cont.).

Combination	Interaction	Mechanism/ Comment	Clinical Significance
	blurred vision, tremor, poor balance, visual hallucination		
MAOI Antidepressant–propranolol	Severe hypertensive crisis may be precipitated	Mechanism ? Probably unopposed α-adrenergic activity in patients receiving sympathomimetic amines, or because of endogenous catecholamines Propranolol contraindicated in patients on MAOI antidepressants or within 2 weeks of stopping such treatment (theoretical consideration)	Yes
Marijuana-propranolol	Inhibits increase in heart rate and systolic blood pressure induced by marijuana May ↓ marijuana-induced reddening of the eyes and learning impairment	Mechanism ? (propranolol blocks β-adrenergic stimulation produced by marijuana)	?

Methyldopa (Aldomet)-propranolol	Hypertensive crisis	α-Methyldopa-norepinephrine (methyldopa metabolite)–mediated vasoconstriction effects are unopposed due to β-blockade Risk may be limited to severely hypertensive patients or those exposed to excessive sympathetic agonists (endogenous or exogenous) Closely monitor for acute blood pressure increases during the combination Treatment: α-adrenergic blocking agents such as phentolamine (Regitine)	?
Narcotic analgesics (morphine, other opiates)–propanolol	Propranolol markedly enhances lethality of toxic doses of morphine in animals	Mechanism ? Use this combination with caution, especially if large doses of one or both drugs are being used	?
Neuromuscular blockers, nondepolarizing group (tubocurarine, etc.) with propanolol	May enhance or counteract the actions of neuromuscular blockers	Mechanism ? Conflicting evidence Monitor patients for respiratory distress during combined therapy	?

(Continued.)

Table 7–1 (cont.).

Combination	Interaction	Mechanism/ Comment	Clinical Significance
Nifedipine–propranolol, atenolol, etc	Pharmacologic effects of both drugs may be enhanced (hypotension or cardiac failure)	Possible synergistic or additive effects Predisposing factors: preexisting left ventricular dysfunction and large doses of β-blocker No specific precautions appear necessary	?
NSAIDs (e.g., indomethacin [Indocin], ibuprofen [Motrin], piroxicam [Feldene])	↓ Therapeutic (antihypertensive and antianginal [?]) effects of β-blockers	Mechanism not established; probably due to NSAIDs inhibiting renal prostaglandin synthesis allowing unopposed pressor systems to produce hypertension Avoid this combination if possible May need a higher dose of β-blockers during combination	Yes
Penicillins, oral (e.g., ampicillin)–atenolol	Therapeutic effects of atenolol may be impaired	Ampicillin impairs GI absorption of atenolol	Yes
	May potentiate anaphylactic reactions of penicillin (case reports)	Decrease intracellular cyclic adenosine monophosphate levels	?

		If an interaction is suspected, consider ↑ dose of atenolol and monitor blood pressure closely	
Phenothiazine-propranolol	(See Table 4–1)		
Phenylephrine-propranolol	Acute hypertensive episode	Propranolol may enhance pressor response to phenylephrine Very limited evidence	?
Phenytoin-propranolol	May ↑ cardiac depressant effects	Additive effect based on theoretical considerations Use this combination with great caution (especially IV use of diphenylhydantoin)	?
Prazosin (Minipress)-propranolol	↑ Postural hypotension produced by prazosin (first-dose response; propranolol may inhibit compensatory cardiovascular response to prozasin-induced hypotension)	Mechanism: ? In patients receiving propranolol, initiate prazosin with conservative doses; taking the initial dose at bedtime may be prudent; otherwise, patients on combined therapy should be advised of chance of postural hypotension developing in early stages of therapy	Yes

(Continued.)

Table 7–1 (cont.).

Combination	Interaction	Mechanism/ Comment	Clinical Significance
Propafenone (Rythmol)-propranolol	May ↑ pharmacologic effect of propranolol	By both decreasing first-pass metabolism and reducing systemic clearance of β-blockers that undergo hepatic elimination	Yes
Propoxyphene (Darvon)-propranolol	May ↑ the bioavailability of propranolol	Propoxyphene may inhibit hepatic metabolism of propranolol	?
Quinidine–propranolol, atenolol	Pharmacologic effects of propranolol, etc. may be increased May ↑ cardiac depressant effects	Quinidine may inhibit oxidative metabolism of β-blockers Advantage in various cardiac arrhythmias No specific precautions appear necessary	Yes
Rifampin-propranolol	May ↓ propranolol plasma levels and pharmacologic effects	Rifampin may enhance hepatic metabolism of propranolol Interaction is of rapid onset with long-lasting effect (may need 3–4 wk washout period for enzyme induction effect to disappear)	Yes

Salicylates (e.g., aspirin)-propanolol	May ↓ hypotensive effect of propranolol	Salicylates may inhibit biosynthesis of prostaglandins involved in antihypertensive activity of propranolol Very limited information: single-dose studies only (multiple doses, long-term effect?)	
Sulfonylureas (e.g., chlorpropamide [Diabinese], tolbutamide [Orinase]) with propranolol	Propranolol may decrease, prolong, or have no effect on hypoglycemic effects of sulfonylureas	Mechanism ? Monitor blood glucose during combination	?
Terbutaline (Brethine, Bricanyl) with nonspecific β-blockers (e.g., propranolol)	May impair the broncho-dilation effects of terbutaline	Antagonistic effects Any β-blocker should be used with caution in asthmatics Practolol appears to be reasonably safe in this combination	Yes
Theophyllines (e.g., aminophylline, theophylline)-propranolol	Reduce elimination of theophylline	Propranolol inhibits hepatic metabolism of theophylline	Yes
	Reduce effects of one or both medications	Antagonistic effects Monitor plasma theophylline levels during and after coadministration Selective β-blockers may be preferred	
Verapamil–propranolol, atenolol	(See Table 2-4)		

Complete suppression of tremor is rarely achieved. For migraine prophylaxis in adults the initial dosage is 80 mg/day in divided doses, which is gradually titrated upward if necessary to 160 to 240 mg/day. Optimal therapeutic response may be achieved within 4 to 6 weeks after the initiation of drug treatment. The drug should be discontinued gradually.

In cases of severe cocaine toxicity, IV propranolol may be useful, with 1-mg doses injected every minute for up to 8 minutes.

Administration. Propranolol is usually administered orally in divided doses before meals and at bedtime. However, the extended-release capsules are usually administered once a day.

Preparations

Propranolol hydrochloride
  Oral capsules, extended-release (*Inderal LA*)
    60 mg, 80 mg, 120 mg, 160 mg
Solution
  20 mg/5 mL, 40 mg/5 mL
  Tablets (*Inderal*)
    10 mg, 20 mg, 40 mg, 60 mg, 80 mg, 90 mg

ATENOLOL

Atenolol is a selective β_1-adrenergic blocking agent. The selectivity for β_1-adrenergic receptors is lost when daily doses exceed approximately 100 mg. The blockade of β_1-adrenergic receptors produces negative chronotropic and inotropic activity. Doses less than 100 mg/day of atenolol have minimal effect on bronchial airway resistance.

Pharmacokinetics

Absorption. Approximately 50% to 60% of an orally administered dose of atenolol is rapidly absorbed from the GI tract. The onset of drug action usually occurs approximately 1 hour after oral administration.

Distribution. Atenolol is widely distributed throughout most body tissues and fluids with the exception of the brain and cerebrospinal fluid (CSF). It readily crosses the placenta and is distributed into human breast milk.

Elimination. Atenolol has a half-life of approximately 6 to 7 hours which may be increased up to 27 hours in patients with renal impairment. The drug is excreted in the urine and feces.

Uses

Atenolol is used for the management of hypertension and angina. It is also used to treat lithium-induced tremor and akathisia.

Cautions

In many cases adverse effects may be attenuated by a reduction in dosage. Abrupt withdrawal should be avoided since it may exacerbate angina or precipitate myocardial infarction.

Cardiovascular Effects. Bradycardia, hypertension, and AV block may also occur.

CNS Effects. Atenolol may produce fatigue, dizziness, depression, lethargy, drowsiness, and vertigo. There may be emotional lability and impairment of short-term memory.

GI Effects. Diarrhea and nausea may occur in some patients.

Other Adverse Effects. Rashes, wheezing, and dyspnea may occur.

Precautions and Contraindications. When atenolol is administered to patients with inadequate cardiac function, there may be precipitation of congestive heart failure. The drug should be avoided in patients with bronchospastic disease because it may inhibit bronchodilation. The drug may mask the symptoms associated with hypoglycemia and hyperthyroidism, and should therefore be used with caution in patients with diabetes mellitus or hyperthyroidism. Atenolol is contraindicated in patients with significant cardiac arrhythmias such as first degree or greater AV block and sinus bradycardia. It should not be used in patients with overt cardiac failure.

Pregnancy, Fertility, and Lactation. There are limited studies regarding the use of atenolol in pregnant women. To date these suggest that when used in the third trimester, atenolol is not associated with significant complications. However, animal studies have shown that in doses ranging from 12 to 25 times the usual human dosages, there may be an increase in embryonal and fetal resorption. There is no evidence of impaired fertility. Atenolol is distributed into breast milk. Thus, caution should be exercised when administering atenolol to nursing women, and these women should be encouraged to use formula.

Acute Toxicity

Manifestations. Overdosage may produce bradycardia, hypotension, cardiac failure, and bronchospasm. Hypoglycemia may occur.

Treatment. The stomach should be emptied via gastric lavage. Symptomatic bradycardia may be treated with atropine; if this is inadequate, isoproterenol may be used. Severe hypotension may be treated with dobutamine, dopamine, or epinephrine. Bronchospasm may be treated with aminophylline, atropine, isoproterenol, or other β_2-agonists. Heart failure may be treated with a diuretic, a cardiac glycoside, and oxygen.

Drug Interactions. Caution should be exercised when other hypotensive agents are coadministered because of the possibility that their hypotensive effects may be potentiated.

Dosage and Administration

Dosage. The dose of atenolol should be titrated to the patient's need and tolerance. If it is discontinued this should be done gradually. The usual dose is 50 mg once a day for the treatment of akathisia or lithium-induced tremor. Dosage should be modified in cases of impaired renal function. Final dosages may be 100 to 200 mg once a day.

Administration. Atenolol is administered orally on a once-a-day basis.

Preparations

Atenolol (*Tenormin*)
  Oral tablets
    50 mg, 100 mg

Skeletal Muscle Relaxant

DANTROLENE SODIUM

Pharmacology

Dantrolene affects skeletal muscle directly. It appears to act by reducing the release of calcium from the sarcoplasmic reticulum. This results in a decreased calcium flux response of the muscle to the action potential, and therefore a decreased muscle contraction.

Pharmacokinetics

Absorption. On average approximately 35% of the oral dose is absorbed from the GI tract. Therapeutic blood concentrations vary widely among individuals, but reportedly range from 100 to 600 ng/mL.

Elimination. Dantrolene is metabolized in the liver to a less active form.

Uses

Dantrolene sodium has been used successfully to treat patients with NMS and malignant hyperthermia.

Cautions

Adverse effects occur commonly. The most common effect is muscle weakness often manifested by slurred speech, enuresis, and drooling. Other common effects include drowsiness, diarrhea, lightheadedness, dizziness, nausea, malaise, and fatigue. These effects are usually transient, lasting approximately 4 days after the initiation of oral therapy. They appear to be dose-related.

Hepatic Effects. Oral dantrolene has been associated with abnormal liver function tests, in particular, increased serum AST, ALT, alkaline phosphatase, LDH, and total serum bilirubin. If detected early, these will return to normal with cessation of drug use. Fatal and nonfatal hepatitis have occurred in patients receiving dantrolene and appear to be idiosyncratic reactions. In most cases, nausea, vomiting, anorexia, and abdominal discomfort precede the onset of hepatitis.

GI Effects. In addition to diarrhea, nausea, anorexia, vomiting, gastric irritation, abdominal cramps, constipation, and GI bleeding have been reported. These symptoms usually respond to a reduction in dosage or discontinuation of the drug.

Nervous System Effects. Manifestations may include speech disturbance, visual disturbances, depression, confusion, and hallucinations, along with the exacerbation or precipitation of seizures.

Urogenital Effects. These may include urinary frequency, incontinence, nocturia, difficulty initiating urination, and urinary retention, individually or severally.

Precautions and Contraindications. Serum AST and ALT, alkaline phosphatase, and total serum bilirubin concentrations should be determined prior to oral dantrolene therapy, and repeated periodically during therapy or whenever symptoms of hepatitis occur. If liver function test abnormalities occur, dantrolene should usually be discontinued. The risk of hepatotoxicity is greater in females, patients older than 35 years of age, and in those receiving other drugs concomitantly (especially estrogens). Patients who engage in potentially hazardous activities requiring mental alertness should be cautioned about possible weakness, dizziness, or drowsiness. Dantrolene may produce difficulty in swallowing, and care should be used at mealtimes to minimize the risk of choking and dysphagia.

Dosage and Administration

Dosage. The dosage for NMS ranges from 0.8 to 10 mg/kg body weight per day. The initial dosage should be 263 mg/kg/day. The oral dosage has ranged from 50 to 200 mg/day. Hepatic toxicity may occur with doses above 10 mg/kg/day.

Administration. Dantrolene may be administered orally, by IV injection, or by IV infusion.

Preparations

Dantrolene sodium
- Oral capsules (*Dantrium*)
  - 25 mg, 50 mg, 100 mg
- Parenteral, for injection (*Dantrium Intravenous*)
  - 20 mg

Alcohol Deterrent

DISULFIRAM

Pharmacology

Disulfiram produces a hypersensitivity to alcohol by inhibiting the enzymatic oxidation of acetaldehyde to acetate. This process is part of the normal metabolism of alcohol in the liver.

Disulfiram produces an irreversible inhibition of enzyme activity by competing with nicotinamide adenine dinucleotide for aldehyde dehydrogenase. After the administration of disulfiram the ingestion of small amounts of alcohol may result in blood levels of acetaldehyde that are 5 to 10 times those found during normal alcohol metabolism. It is believed that the high blood concentrations of acetaldehyde are responsible for the disulfiram-alcohol reaction; however, it has also been suggested that a toxic quaternary ammonium compound may be responsible.

Tolerance does not occur to disulfiram. Sensitivity to the ingestion of alcohol increases with prolonged administration of disulfiram.

Pharmacokinetics

Absorption. While disulfiram is rapidly absorbed from the liver, up to 12 hours may be necessary before the effects of the drug become apparent. Toxic reactions may occur up to 1 to 2 weeks following the last dose of disulfiram.

Elimination. Eighty percent to 95% of the administered dose is absorbed; the remainder is excreted unmetabolized in the feces.

Uses

Disulfiram is used as an adjunct in the management of alcohol dependence to deter alcohol consumption. The best results occur in highly motivated patients when the drug is used in conjunction with other forms of therapy. The long-term efficacy of disulfiram has not been established; however, it appears that without appropriate supportive therapy and motivation, disulfiram is unlikely to be of major benefit. After ingesting as little as 15 mL of 100 proof whiskey or its equivalent, patients who are consuming disulfiram will experience severe side effects which may require prompt medical attention and usually develop within 5 to 15 minutes after alcohol ingestion. Prior to initiating treatment with disulfiram, the patient should undergo a complete physical examination and receive an adequate explanation of the nature of the alcohol-disulfiram interaction. In particular, the patient should be cautioned against ingesting alcohol and alcohol-containing foods or medicines, not only during the period of alcohol administration, but for 2 weeks after discontinuation of disulfiram.

Cautions

Disulfiram-Alcohol Reaction. After the ingestion of alcohol in subjects consuming disulfiram, the reaction may persist anywhere from several hours to as short as 30 minutes. The intensity and duration of the reaction are alcohol dose–dependent, but are also influenced by the dosage of disulfiram and individual variation. Symptoms of the reaction consist of flushing, throbing in the head and neck, including headache, nausea, vomiting, sweating, thirst, dyspnea, chest pain, palpitations, hyperventilation, tachycardia, hypotension, anxiety, weakness, syncope, vertigo, blurred vision, and confusion.

Mild reactions, which are associated with blood concentrations of 5 to 10 mg/dL of blood alcohol, may be followed by sound sleep and complete recovery. However, with higher blood alcohol concentrations, in particular, those greater than 125 to 250 mg/dL, there may a progression to respiratory depression, cardiovascular collapse, arrhythmias, myocardial infarction, acute congestive heart failure, unconsciousness, seizures, and death. Most fatal interactions have occurred when the patient was consuming greater than 500 mg/day of disulfiram and had ingested more than two alcoholic drinks.

Treatment of the disulfiram-alcohol reaction is supportive and symptomatic; however, these reactions should be managed in facilities with access to emergency equipment and drugs, since arrhythmias and severe hypotension may occur. Severe reactions should be treated like shock; respiration should be assisted with oxygen; and plasma or electrolyte solutions may be given to maintain circulation. Pressor agents may be required for hypotension.

Other Adverse Effects. Adverse effects may develop in the absence of alcohol consumption; these are most likely to occur during the first 2 weeks of therapy. Most commonly, they consist of impotence, fatigue, drowsiness, headache, acneiform or allergic dermatitis, and a metallic or garliclike aftertaste. Skin eruptions may be treated with antihistamine therapy. Less commonly, vertigo, irritability, abnormal gait, insomnia, slurred speech, disorientation, confusion, and personality changes have been reported. Also uncommon are tonoclonic seizures, peripheral neuropathy, polyneuritis, optic neuritis, delirium, bizarre behavior, and psychoses.

Disulfiram may aggravate preexisting EEG abnormalities. Hepatitis and blood dyscrasias have been reported. Patients receiving disulfiram therapy should be cautioned to avoid alcohol-containing products such as cough syrups, vinegars, elixirs, and sauces. Likewise, the external application of alcohol liniments or lotions, including aftershave and rubbing alcohol lotions, may be sufficient to produce a disulfiram-alcohol reaction. Furthermore, patients should be cautioned that the disulfiram-alcohol reaction may occur several weeks after the discontinuation of disulfiram. Patients should fully understand the nature of the disulfiram interaction and its manifestations. Close relatives should also be advised of the risks and manifestations of the reaction. The patient should be advised to carry identifying information regarding his or her use of disulfiram.

Baseline and follow-up transaminase determinations are recommended every 2 weeks and a complete blood count obtained every 6 months in patients receiving disulfiram, because of hypersensitivity hepatitis and blood dyscrasias.

Disulfiram is contraindicated in patients with alcohol intoxication, cardiovascular disease, and psychoses. It should be given with caution to those patients with diabetes mellitus, hypothyroidism, seizures or structural CNS damage, chronic or acute nephritis, hepatic cirrhosis, or abnormal EEG results.

Acute Toxicity

Symptoms of toxicity due to acute ingestion include GI upset, vomiting, abnormal EEG findings, altered consciousness, hallucinations, drowsiness, incoordination, speech impairment, and coma. Gastric lavage may be helpful in addition to supportive therapy.

Drug Interactions

Concomitant use of disulfiram and oral anticoagulants should be avoided if possible. Studies in healthy subjects indicate that disulfiram augments the hypoprothrombinemic effect and increases plasma levels of warfarin.

Disulfiram may inhibit the hepatic metabolism of benzodiazepines that undergo oxidation and possibly increase the CNS depressant effects. CNS stimulation and the cardiovascular effects of caffeine may be increased by disulfiram, possibly due to inhibition of caffeine hepatic metabolism. Taking alcohol, even in small quantities, after the administration of disulfiram produces an extremely unpleasant syndrome characterized by a generalized pruritic macular skin rash, flushing, nausea, vertigo, blurred vision, tachycardia, dyspnea, and hypotension. This effect is due to an increase of acetaldehyde in the blood. The use of ethanol-containing local applications and oral liquid pharmaceutical preparations may also produce a reaction.

Both disulfiram and isoniazid may inhibit the metabolic paths for dopamine (inhibit β-hydroxylase and monoamine oxidase, respectively). The inhibition results in increased methylated metabolites of dopamine (by the catechol-*o*-methyltransferase pathway), which may be responsible for the adverse mental changes and coordination problems. Preliminary reports described psychotic episodes and confusional states in patients using metronidazole-disulfiram combined therapy. Although these reports involved small numbers of patients, it seems likely that the interaction is clinically significant. Several studies and case reports have demonstrated that concomitant disulfiram administration significantly increases serum phenytoin levels which may lead to phenytoin toxicity. The rise was rapid, occurring within 4 hours of the first dose of disulfiram, and continued to rise for several days after disulfiram was stopped. Disulfiram should be used under close supervision in patients receiving phenytoin with serum levels determined prior to and during disulfiram therapy. The concomitant administration of disulfiram and a tricyclic antidepressant may result in acute brain syndrome, but a cause-and-effect relationship between the drug interaction and the symptom has not been established.

Amitriptyline is said to enhance the alcohol reaction in patients taking disulfiram. Disulfiram inhibits both the hydroxylation and demethylation pathways of theophylline metabolism. Thus, coadministration of disulfiram and theophylline may increase the pharmacologic and toxic effects of the latter. Disulfiram should not be administered with paraldehyde because paraldehyde is depolymerized to acetaldehyde in the liver. Disulfiram may impair the deposition of acetaldehyde by inhibition of acetaldehyde dehydrogenase. The interactions between disulfiram and other commonly used medications are shown in Table 7–2.

Dosage and Administration

Dosage. Disulfiram is initially given as 250 to 500 mg every morning for the first 1 to 2 weeks, then decreased to 250 mg/day. The administration may be switched to bedtime if daytime seda-

Table 7–2.
Drug Interactions With Disulfiram

Combination	Interaction	Mechanism/ Comment	Clinical Significance
Anticoagulants, oral, e.g., Warfarin (Coumadin)	↑ Anticoagulant effect (↑ hypoprothrombinemic effect and ↑ plasma levels of warfarin)	Mechanism unknown Avoid combination if possible	Yes
Benzodiazepines (oxidation) e.g., alprazolam (Xanax), chlordiazepoxide (Librium), diazepam (Valium)	May ↑ CNS depressant action	Disulfiram may inhibit metabolism of benzodiazepines that undergo oxidation (oxazepam, lorazepam, etc. metabolized by glucoronidation were not affected by disulfiram coadministration) If ↑ CNS depressant effects occur, benzodiazepine dose may need to be decreased	Yes
Caffeine	May ↑ cardiovascular and CNS stimulation effects of caffeine	Disulfiram may inhibit hepatic metabolism of caffeine	?
Ethanol (Alcohol)	Generalized pruritic macular rash, flushing, nausea, vertigo, dyspnea, tachycardia, etc	Disulfiram inhibits aldehyde dehydrogenase, causing accumulation of acetaldehyde Using ethanol-containing local	Yes

(Continued.)

		applications and oral liquid pharmaceutical preparations may result in mild reactions Death has been reported The combination should be undertaken with careful observation	
Isoniazid	Acute behavioral and coordination changes	Mechanism unknown possibly excess dopaminergic activity Use the combination with caution Disulfiram alone has been reported to result in acute organic brain syndrome	?
Metronidazole (Flagyl)	Confusion, psychotic episode	Mechanism unknown	Yes
Paraldehyde	May impair depostion of acetaldehyde	Inhibition of acetaldehyde dehydrogenase Theoretical considerations and animal studies indicate that interaction may be clinically significant	?
Perphenazine (PPZ), oral	↓ Plasma PPZ concentration and pharmacologic effect	Disulfiram activates hepatic metabolism of PPZ (to inactive metabolites) Use parenteral PPZ (avoids first-pass effect in the liver) if disulfiram is given at the same time	?

Table 7–2 (cont.).

Combination	Interaction	Mechanism/ Comment	Clinical Significance
Phenytoin (Dilantin)	↑ Serum phenytoin levels and may evoke phenytoin toxicity Rapid onset (within several hours after coadministration) and prolonged effect	Disulfiram inhibits hepatic metabolism of phenytoin Disulfiram ↓ elimination rate of phenytoin by noncompetitive mechanisms If combined treatment is necessary, ↓ phenytoin dosage and monitor phenytoin levels regularly	Yes
Tricyclic antidepressants (TCAs)	Acute organic brain syndrome ↑ TCA bioavailability	Mechanism unknown (↑ dopamine?) Disulfiram may inhibit hepatic metabolism of TCAs	?
Theophyllines (e.g., aminophylline)	↑ Pharmacologic and toxic effects of theophylines	Disulfiram inhibits theophylline metabolism (both hydroxylation and demethylation pathways)	Yes

tion is a problem. Maintenance dosages may range as low as 125 or as high as 500 mg/day. Dosage should not exceed 500 mg/day. Daily administration is continued until abstinence has been well established.

Administration. Disulfiram is administered orally. It may be administered as either a tablet or a suspension of 1% disulfiram, 0.25% methylcellulose, and 10% orange juice in distilled water. This preparation is stable for up to 6 months if refrigerated between 2° and 8°C, and protected from light.

Disulfiram should not be administered until the patient has abstained from alcohol for at least 12 hours and should not be administered without the patient's knowledge.

Preparations

Disulfiram (*Antabuse*)
  Oral tablets
    250 mg, 500 mg

Sedative-Hypnotic

CHLORAL HYDRATE

Chloral hydrate is a sedative-hypnotic with an incompletely understood mechanism of action. It is an effective hypnotic, and in higher doses can be used for general anesthesia; however, it produces concurrent respiratory depression.

Pharmacokinetics

Absorption. Chloral hydrate is rapidly absorbed from the GI tract following oral or rectal administration. Oral administration of chloral hydrate usually produces sleep within 30 to 60 minutes of administration. The hypnotic effects last approximately 4 to 8 hours.

Distribution. Chloral hydrate and its active metabolite trichloroethanol are distributed widely in body fluids including blood and CSF; however, no significant quantities are distributed into human breast milk.

Elimination. Chloral hydrate is metabolized both in the liver and in erythrocytes. The active metabolite trichloroethanol is formed by alcohol dehydrogenase. This active metabolite has a half-life of 8 to 11 hours. Inactive metabolites are excreted in the urine and a lesser amount in the feces.

Uses

Chloral hydrate is used principally as a hypnotic for short-term treatment of insomnia. It loses much of its efficacy for sleep induction and sleep maintenance when treatment exceeds 2 weeks. Chloral hydrate is also effective in preventing the development of alcohol withdrawal symptoms.

Cautions

GI Effects. Gastric irritation is the most common GI effect of chloral hydrate. Its usual manifestations include nausea, vomiting, and diarrhea. These may be minimized by diluting the oral solution or by administering the capsules with larger quantities of fluids.

Nervous Systems Effects. Occasionally, patients may develop somnambulism. There may be paradoxical excitement, disorientation, or incoherence. Rarely, there may be paranoid behavior, confusion, dizziness, headache, and hallucinations.

Precautions and Contraindications. Patients should be cautioned about engaging in hazardous activities or in activities that require mental alertness, such as operating machinery or driving a motor vehicle. Caution should be exercised in patients with hepatic, renal, or respiratory impairment. The drug should also be used cautiously in patients with gastric or duodenal ulcers or gastritis or esophagitis.

Pregnancy, Fertility, and Lactation. Chloral hydrate crosses the placenta and accumulates in the fetus. Fetal effects are unknown; therefore, caution should be exercised when administering this drug to pregnant women. Withdrawal symptoms may occur in neonates. Small quantities of chloral hydrate and its active metabolite may be found in breast milk; these do not appear to cause clinically significant effects in the newborn.

Chronic Toxicity

Tolerance and physical dependence may develop when the drug is taken for longer than 2 weeks. Symptoms of dependence include dose escalation, drowsiness, hangover, lethargy, slurring of speech, nystagmus, incoordination, and tremulousness. Sudden withdrawal can precipitate a withdrawal syndrome which includes hallucinations and delirium tremens. For this reason sudden withdrawal should be avoided. Furthermore, prolonged administration may be associated with gastritis, skin eruptions, or renal damage. Attempts to decrease the dose are associated with insomnia, which may persist for a few days.

Acute Toxicity

Manifestations. Chloral hydrate overdosage may produce coma, respiratory depression, and cardiac arrhythmias. There may be hypothermia, hypotension, an absence of reflexes, muscle flaccidity, and miosis. Hepatic and renal function may be impaired. Death usually results from hypotension or respiratory failure. The usual lethal dose in adults is 10 g. Treatment consists of general supportive approaches, including maintaining adequate airway, respiration, body temperature, and circulation. Gastric lavage may be performed. Peritoneal or hemodialysis may enhance the elimination of trichloroethanol.

Drug Interactions

CNS depressants and alcohol may produce additive CNS depression along with facial flushing, dysphoria, tachycardia, headache, and palpitations. Additive CNS depression may occur with other CNS depressants. When chloral hydrate is administered within 24 hours of the administration of IV furosemide, there may be diaphoresis, fluctuations in blood pressure, flushing, and general malaise. There is some evidence that hypoalbuminemia may increase the likelihood of symptoms from this interaction. Chloral hydrate may potentiate the anticoagulant effects of warfarin by displacing warfarin from its binding sites on plasma albumin. Since this effect is usually small and fleeting, chloral hydrate appears safe to use with warfarin. However, benzodiazepines do not appear to affect anticoagulant control at all and are very safe alternatives. The interactions between chloral hydrate and other commonly used medications are shown in Table 7–3.

Dosage and Administration

Dosage. The dosage should be titrated to the individual's needs and tolerance. The usual hypnotic dose for an adult is 500 mg to

1 g given 15 to 30 minutes before bedtime. For children, the usual hypnotic dose is 50 mg/kg.

Administration. Chloral hydrate may be administered either orally or rectally. When administered as an oral capsule or solution, it should be taken with a full glass of water or other liquids, such as fruit juice or ginger ale, to dilute the chloral hydrate.

Preparations

Chloral hydrate is a schedule C-IV drug.

Chloral hydrate
- Oral capsules (*Noctec*)
  - 250 mg, 500 mg
- Solution (*Noctec Syrup*)
  - 250 mg/5 mL, 500 mg/5 mL
- Rectal suppositories
  - 325 mg (*Aquachloral Supprettes*), 500 mg (*Chloral Hydrate Suppositories*), 650 mg (*Aquachloral Supprettes*)

THYROID HORMONE

LIOTHYRONINE SODIUM

Liothyronine sodium is the synthetically prepared sodium salt of the levorotatory isomer of 3, 3′, 5-triiodothyronine (T_3). Its principle pharmacologic effect is to enhance cellular metabolic rates. It also affects cell growth and differentiation.

Pharmacokinetics

Ninety-five percent of an orally administered dose is absorbed from the GI tract. It is not highly bound by thyroxine-binding globulin, but is 99% bound to serum proteins. The usual plasma half-life is 1 to 2 days.

Uses

T_3 is used adjunctively with other antidepressant medications in the treatment of refractory major depression. Though its efficacy is controversial, it may be especially helpful in women with refractory depression.

Table 7–3.
Drug Interactions With Chloral Hydrate

Combination	Interaction	Mechanism/ Comment	Clinical Significance
Alcohol or other CNS depressants	↑ Hypnotic and CNS depressant effects of chloral hydrate Flushing, tachycardia, headache also occur Performance of motor tasks is more impaired	Synergistic effects (↑ reduction of chloral hydrate to trichloroethanol through metabolic competition in alcohol dehydrogenase–mediated process) Patients at significant risk of disulfiram reaction should avoid concomitant use	Yes
Anticoagulants, oral, e.g., dicumarol, warfarin (Coumadin)	May temporarily ↑ anticoagulant effects	Trichloroacetic acid, a metabolite of chloral hydrate, displaces warfarin from its binding sites Approach this combination with caution Benzodiazepines are safe alternatives for patients on anticoagulant therapy	?

Furosemide, IV (Lasix)	Transient diaphoresis, flushed skin, labile blood pressure, nausea, feeling of uneasiness	Mechanism unknown Observe closely for interaction effect within 24 hr after coadministration Reaction to oral furosemide?	?
Phenytoin (Dilantin)	May ↓ phenytoin therapeutic action	↑ Hepatic metabolism of phenytoin (↑ elimination) A single, small study proposed interaction	?

Patients with mood disorders should have their thyroid function checked. Hyper- or hypothyroidism can simulate primary mood disorders. Furthermore, even subclinical thyroid imbalance may be associated with treatment-refractory mood disorders. Correcting such a subclinical state is separate from the above-described use of liothyronine as a treatment adjunct with euthyroid patients.

Cautions

Adverse effects result from overdosage and are the signs and symptoms of hyperthyroidism. These may include weight loss, palpitations, nervousness, increased appetite, abdominal cramps, diarrhea, sweating, tachycardia, increased pulse and blood pressure, angina, cardiac arrhythmias, tremor, insomnia, headache, heat intolerance, fever, and menstrual irregularities.

Patients receiving thyroid hormone should be monitored closely and thyroid functions checked periodically by appropriate laboratory studies. Thyroid agents should be used with caution and in low doses in patients with coronary artery disease or other cardiovascular disease, including hypertension.

Dosage and Administration

Dosage. For adjunctive treatment of depression, liothyronine is usually given in a dosage of 25 to 50 μg/day for 10 days. If no improvement in depression is evident after this time, the trial can be considered a failure and the drug discontinued.

Administration. Liothyronine sodium is administered orally.

Preparations

Liothyronine sodium (*Cytomel*)
  Oral tablets
    5 μg, 25 μg, 50 μg

ANTIPARKINSONIAN AGENTS 8

GENERAL STATEMENT

Antimuscarinics and dopaminergic agonists are the two classes of drugs commonly used by psychiatrists for treatment or prevention of the extrapyramidal side effects induced by neuroleptics.

Anticholinergic Adverse Effects

Most adverse effects are usually reversible when drug therapy is discontinued. The frequency and severity of adverse effects are generally dose-related.

Adverse reactions frequently associated with the use of anticholinergic agents include dry mouth, blurred vision, photophobia, urinary hesitancy and retention, palpitations, tachycardia, and constipation. Other effects include loss of taste, headache, nervousness, weakness, drowsiness, insomnia, dizziness, flushing, nausea, vomiting, and a bloated feeling. Some individuals may exhibit an unusual sensitivity and manifest toxic symptoms at the usual therapeutic dosages. These may range up to complete disorientation or delirium. The risk of hyperthermia is increased with elevated ambient temperature and in those patients manifesting fever. Because of the tendency to produce drowsiness and blurred vision the patient should be warned about the hazards associated with activities that require mental alertness or visual acuity (such as operating a motor vehicle, or other machinery).

Antimuscarinic anticholinergic agents should be used with caution in geriatric patients and in children since both populations may be at greater risk for the development of delirium and other adverse effects.

AMANTADINE HYDROCHLORIDE

Chemistry

Amantadine is used in the treatment of parkinsonian syndrome and is structurally unrelated to other antiparkinsonian agents.

Amantadine is the only dopamine agonist commonly used by psychiatrists.

Pharmacology

Amantadine may have mild anticholinergic activity. Its primary effect is thought to be potentiation of dopaminergic neurotransmission in the central nervous system (CNS), possibly by blocking reuptake of dopamine into the presynaptic neuron, thus causing dopamine to accumulate in the presynaptic cleft of dopaminergic neurons in the basal ganglia. It may, however, also directly stimulate postsynaptic receptors, and may cause the release of catecholamines from nerve storage sites.

Pharmacokinetics

Absorption. Amantadine is well absorbed from the gastrointestinal (GI) tract. Steady-state blood levels after oral administration are achieved 4 to 5 days after the initiation of therapy.

Elimination. The elimination half-life of amantadine in young adults is 14 hours, and is about 29 hours in the elderly. It is excreted unchanged in the urine and does not appear to be removed by hemodialysis.

Uses

Amantadine hydrochloride is useful in the treatment of neuroleptic-induced extrapyramidal, parkinsonian effects. Its antiparkinsonian effects tend to be weaker than the effects of anticholinergic antiparkinsonian medications. It can be useful for patients unable to tolerate anticholinergic side effects.Amantadine may be administered concurrently with anticholinergic, antiparkinsonian agents.

Cautions

Nervous System Effects. Adverse effects are usually reversible and dose-related. They may appear within a few hours or days after initiation of treatment and likewise may occur a few hours after an increase in drug dosage. Most commonly, insomnia, dizziness, nervousness, and impaired concentration may occur and are seen in 5% to 10% of patients. Side effects usually disappear with discontinuation of drug. Irritability, depression, ataxia, anxiety, confusion, hallucinations, and headache have been reported in 1% to 5% of patients. Fatigue, slurred speech, weakness, and psychosis have been reported in less than 1%. Patients with an active seizure disorder may experience an increase in their seizure frequency. Orthostatic hypotension is not uncommon.

Livido Reticularis. Livido reticularis is a frequent adverse effect in patients taking amantadine. It usually occurs in the legs and diminishes with elevation of the extremities. It occurs in 1% to 5% of patients, usually appearing within the first few months of treatment. It will subside with discontinuation of amantadine, and may resolve even during continued treatment.

GI Effects. Nausea may occur in 10% to 15% of patients. Constipation, dry mouth, anorexia, and vomiting may occur in approximately 1% of patients.

Other Adverse Effects. Edema, congestive heart failure, rash, and visual disturbances occur in less than 1%.

Precautions and Contraindications

Amantadine should be used with caution in patients with liver disease, eczematoid dermatitis, and epilepsy. Because of CNS effects and visual disturbances, patients should be cautioned about operating hazardous machinery or engaging in activities which require sustained concentration.

Drug Interactions

Drugs With Anticholinergic Activity. Administration of amantadine to patients receiving anticholinergic drugs may result in increased anticholinergic effects (Table 8–1). This is rare.

CNS Stimulants. To avoid the possibility of additive CNS stimulant effects, amantadine should be used with caution in patients already receiving CNS stimulant drugs.

Dosage and Administration

Dosage. The usual dosage is 100 mg twice a day. Occasionally patients may not respond at 200 mg/day and will benefit from a dosage increase to 400 mg/day in divided doses. However, a dosage greater than 200 mg/day should be accompanied by close physician observation.

Administration. Amantadine is always administered orally.

Preparations

Amantadine hydrochloride
  Oral capsules (*Symadine, Symmetrel*)
    100 mg

Solution (*Symmetrel Syrup*)
50 mg/5 mL
Tablets (*Symmetrel*)
100 mg

BENZTROPINE MESYLATE

Pharmacology

The anticholinergic effects of benztropine are about equal to those of atropine. The full effects of benztropine may not be seen until 2 to 3 days after treatment has been initiated owing to the cumulative nature of the drug effects.

Uses

Benztropine may be used for the relief of parkinsonian signs and symptoms associated with antipsychotic agents.

Cautions

Adverse Effects. Adverse effects are predominantly antihistaminic and anticholinergic. In moderate doses they may consist of tachycardia, dryness of the mouth, nervousness, blurred vision, and nausea. As the dose increases, side effects include confusion, excitement, weakness, urinary retention, constipation, listlessness, depression, visual hallucinations, and hyperesthesia of the extremities. Management usually consists of lowering the dosage.

Precautions and Contraindications

Benztropine should be used with caution in patients in whom anticholinergic or antihistaminic effects may be undesirable. Because of the cumulative effects, close monitoring should be used at the initiation of treatment since a toxic psychosis or worsening of mental symptoms may occur. Those patients receiving neuroleptics with strong anticholinergic effects should be particularly cognizant about alerting their physicians to the development of problematic anticholinergic effects, such as constipation and urinary difficulties.

Dosage and Administration

Dosage. For the symptomatic relief of extrapyramidal symptoms induced from the administration of a neuroleptic, 1 to 2 mg administered 2 to 3 times a day usually provides relief within 1 to 2 days. Dosages exceeding 8 mg/day should be avoided. Acute extrapyramidal symptoms are generally transient and the need for ongoing anticholinergic agents should be assessed after the first 1 to 2 weeks of therapy.

For the treatment of acute dystonic reaction, 1 to 2 mg of benztropine may be given intramuscularly (IM) or intravenously (IV) followed by 1 to 2 mg orally twice a day to prevent recurrence.

Administration. Benztropine is administered as a parenteral preparation or orally. Parenteral administration is used most commonly for emergency situations such as acute dystonic reactions, when a rapid response is desired. Benztropine may be administered IV. However, there is no significant difference between IV and IM administration and the IV route is rarely used.

Preparations

Benztropine mesylate (*Cogentin*)
  Oral tablets
    0.5 mg, 1.0 mg, 2.0 mg
  Parenteral injection
    1 mg/mL

BIPERIDEN HYDROCHLORIDE
BIPERIDEN LACTATE

Uses

Biperiden is used for the relief of parkinsonian signs and symptoms induced by antipsychotic agents.

Cautions

Adverse Effects. Adverse effects are mainly an extension of the anticholinergic effects (see the General Statement for additional details). Dry mouth and blurred vision are common, as are GI disturbances, drowsiness, and dizziness. Mental confusion, disorientation, agitation, and urinary retention are less commonly seen.

Parenteral administration may produce transient postural hypotension, impaired coordination, and transient euphoria. This may be more common with IV administration.

Table 8–1.
Drug Interactions With Antiparkinsonian Agents

Combination	Interaction	Mechanism/ Comment	Clinical Significance
Amantadine (Symmetrel) + antiparkinsonian anticholinergics, e.g., benztropine, biperiden, orphenadrine (Disipal) trihexyphenidyl	↑ Anticholinergic side effects	Possibly additive or synergistic effects Decrease dose of anticholinergic agent during coadministration of amantadine	?
Amantadine, triamterene (Dyrenium), hydrochlorothiazide (HydroDIURIL)	May increase serum concentration of amantadine and risk for developing toxicity from amantadine	Reduce renal clearance; mechanism unknown Case report: a suspected interaction between amantadine and Dyazide (triamterene + hydrochlorothiazide)	?
Antiparkinsonian anticholinergics (e.g., benztropine, biperiden, cycrimine) + antipsychotics (AP)	Pharmacologic/therapeutic actions of AP could be reduced with centrally acting anticholinergics	Anticholinergics probably antagonize phenothiazines (PTZs) by direct CNS cholinergic pathways; acceleration of PTZ gut metabolism has also been postulated	Yes

Ethopropazine (Parsidol), orphenadrine, procyclidine (Kemadrin), trihexyphenidyl + chlorpromazine, haloperidol. etc.	Amelioration of AP-induced extrapyramidal syndrome (EPS)	EPS most responsive to antiparkinsonian agents are: pseudoparkinsonism, perioral tremor, acute dystonia Short-term (3–4 mo) treatment with benztropine, etc. may suffice to effectively deal with AP-induced parkinsonism Long-term combined therapy may increase risk for developing tardive dyskinesia Additive anticholinergic action from combination may be hazardous in angle-closure glaucoma or in individuals hypersensitive to parasympathetic blockade	
Levodopa-trihexyphenidyl	May reduce therapeutic utility of levodopa	Mechanism unknown Conflicting results; some reports refute finding	?
Monoamine oxidase inhibitor antidepressants	Potentiate action of antiparkinsonian agents	Use combination with caution Dosage of antiparkinsonian drugs may have to be reduced	
Quinidine	↑ Vagolytic effects	Caution should be observed with this combination	?

Precautions and Contraindications

Biperiden should be used with caution in those patients in whom anticholinergic effects are undesirable (see the General Statement about precautions and contraindications associated with anticholinergic agents).

Drug Interactions

Concomitant administration of other anticholinergic effects may be more likely to produce problematic side effects (see Table 7–1).

Dosage and Administration

Dosage. Dosage should be titrated to individual needs. For the treatment of an acute drug-induced dystonic reaction the usual adult dosage is 2 mg IM or by slow IV bolus injection. This may be repeated every 30 minutes to a total of 8 mg/24 hr. The usual adult dosage for the relief of extrapyramidal, parkinsonian symptoms is 2 mg, 1 to 3 times a day.

Administration. Biperiden is administered as the hydrochloride in the oral form, and as the lactate salt when parenterally.

Preparations

Biperiden hydrochloride (*Akineton Hydrochloride*)
- Oral tablets
  - 2 mg

Biperiden lactate (*Akineton Lactate*)
- Parenteral injection
  - 5 mg/mL

TRIHEXYPHENIDYL HYDROCHLORIDE

Pharmacology

Trihexyphenidyl produces more central stimulation than benztropine.

Uses

Trihexyphenidyl is useful in the treatment of neuroleptic-induced extrapyramidal effects.

Cautions

Adverse Effects. Adverse effects of trihexyphenidyl are related to its anticholinergic properties (see the General Statement on anticholinergics for further information).

Adverse effects include dry mouth, blurred vision, nausea, constipation, tachycardia, urinary hesitancy or retention, weakness, and vomiting. There may be restlessness, agitation, confusion, or delirium. Occasionally euphoric symptoms or hallucinations are seen, especially in high dosages. Symptoms of euphoria may account for the fact that trihexyphenidyl is occasionally abused.

Precautions and Contraindications

Trihexyphenidyl should be used with caution in those patients in whom anticholinergic effects would be undesirable.

Dosage and Administration

Dosage. Dosage must be titrated to the individual's needs and response. Dosages usually range from 5 to 15 mg/day.

Administration. Trihexyphenidyl hydrochloride is administered orally. Trihexyphenidyl elixir or conventional tablets may be administered 3 times a day with meals. If a fourth dose is necessary it is frequently given at bedtime. Extended-release capsules of trihexyphenidyl are used in the maintenance phase, but they are not used for the initiation of treatment. They require the establishment of an effective maintenance dosage. This is done by titrating with conventional tablets or elixir. Extended-release capsules may be administered as a single daily morning dose or in two doses every 12 hours. Extended-release capsules may be substituted for the conventional tablets on a milligram-per-milligram basis, once the daily dosage has been established.

Preparations

Trihexyphenidyl hydrochloride
- Oral capsules, extended-release (*Artane Sequels*)
  - 5 mg
- Elixir (*Artane*)
  - 2 mg/5 mL
- Tablets (*Artane, Trixhexane, Trixhexy*)
  - 2 mg, 5 mg

ANTIHISTAMINES 9

Pharmacology

Histamine is a physiologically active substance that binds to H_1 and H_2 receptors. It affects the cardiovascular system, bronchial tree, and stimulates salivary, gastric, lacrimal, and bronchial secretions. Through its ability to stimulate nerve endings, it can cause pruritus. The use of the term *antihistamine* generally describes H_1 receptor antagonists; H_2 antagonists, (e.g., cimetidine, ranitidine) are usually referred to as H_2 *receptor antagonists.* Because an ethylamine group is common to anticholinergic agents and to antihistamines, these drugs manifest some similar activities.

Pharmacokinetics

Absorption. Generally, antihistamines are well absorbed following oral administration. Effects usually begin 15 to 30 minutes after administration, peaking at about 1 hour and lasting a total of 3 to 6 hours. Tolerance to the sedative effects may occur with repeated use.

Uses

Antihistamines, in particular diphenhydramine and doxylamine, are most often used as nighttime sleep inducers owing to their sedative effects. Neuroleptic-induced extrapyramidal symptoms, motion sickness, anorexia nervosa, autism, and anorgasmia (secondary to tricyclic antidepressants) are some of the neuropsychiatric conditions for which antihistamines are used.

Cautions

Adverse effects vary in incidence and severity, but, serious toxicity rarely occurs. Geriatric patients are more likely to develop dizziness, sedation, and hypotension. Mild reactions can usually be managed by dose reduction or by changing to another antihistaminic agent.

CNS Effects. CNS depression is common with antihistamines. Most commonly, sedation ranges from drowsiness to deep sleep. Occasionally, the patient may develop dizziness or disturbed coordination. In light of this, individuals should be cautioned about operating hazardous machinery or driving a motor vehicle because of the drowsiness or dizziness associated with these drugs. Likewise, patients should be cautioned about consumption of alcoholic beverages since these may potentiate the sedative effects.

Children, and rarely adults, receiving antihistamines may experience a paradoxical reaction: excitement, restlessness, tremors, insomnia, nervousness, palpitations, and delirium. This may occasionally progress to seizures.

GI and Hepatic Effects. Adverse effects on the gastrointestinal (GI) system are uncommon. Occasionally, patients will report anorexia after gastric distress, nausea, vomiting, constipation, or diarrhea. The untoward effects may be reduced by administering antihistamines with food or milk.

Anticholinergic Effects of Antihistamines. Antihistamines may induce dry mouth, blurred vision, difficulty in initiating the urinary stream, impotence, vertigo, tinnitus, insomnia, and irritability.

Precautions and Contraindications. Antihistamines having substantial anticholinergic activity should be administered with caution in patients with prostatic hypertrophy, narrow-angle glaucoma, stenosing peptic ulcer, or bladder neck obstruction.

Pregnancy, Fertility, and Lactation. Antihistamines have not been established as being free of teratogenic effects. Therefore, the drugs should not be used unless the potential benefits justify the possible risk to the fetus. The degree of teratogenicity may vary from preparation to preparation. In addition, antihistamines may inhibit lactation and small amounts of the drug may be distributed into breast milk. Because of the possibility of significant central nervous system (CNS) sedation in neonates, the indications for the use of antihistamines in the postpartum period should be carefully weighed against the possible risk to newborns.

Acute Toxicity

Manifestations. Significant overdosage may result in death; infants and young children are at greatest risk. In milder overdose situations, stimulation or sedation are likely. In adults, overdose usually causes CNS depression with drowsiness which progresses in severity to seizures and coma. In adults, there may be cerebral edema. Death may occur from cardiorespiratory collapse. Symptoms of overdose may appear anywhere from 30 minutes to 2 hours after drug ingestion, with death occurring at any time up to 18 hours after ingestion.

Treatment. Treatment of antihistamine overdose is symptomatic with supportive primary care. If emesis cannot be induced, then gastric lavage and administration of activated charcoal should be performed. An endotracheal tube with inflated cuff should be used to prevent aspiration of vomit. Physostigmine may counteract the anticholinergic effects for a brief period of time. Diazepam or other benzodiazepines may be useful in the management of seizures.

Drug Interactions

CNS Depressants. Antihistamines are most likely to enhance the sedative effects of all CNS depressants including alcohol, barbiturates, hypnotics, sedatives, and tranquilizers. Alcohol and other CNS depressants may also enhance the effects of antihistamines. See Table 9–1 for a summary of drug interactions with antihistamines. Patients should be warned that the coadministration of antihistamines and CNS depressants may cause drowsiness and loss of attention and may lead to accidents, particularly with respect to driving or operating hazardous machinery.

Monoamine Oxidase Inhibitors (MAOIs). These drugs may prolong and intensify the anticholinergic effects of antihistamines.

CYPROHEPTADINE

Cyproheptadine is an antihistamine, a serotonin antagonist, and an anticholinergic.

Pharmacokinetics

Absorption. Cyproheptadine is well absorbed following oral administration.

Distribution. Its distribution in body fluids is unknown. Likewise, its metabolism is not fully known.

Elimination. It is metabolized in the liver and excreted in the urine. The excretion of the drug is impaired when renal function is compromised.

Uses

Cyproheptadine is used to treat the early satiety that characterizes refeeding in anorexia nervosa. In the treatment of anorexia nervosa the drug may be more effective in patients who do not have binge eating as an additional feature of their anorexia. It is also used to treat autism. Approximately one third of autistic patients respond to cyproheptadine. Cyproheptadine may be effective in the management of inhibited male and female orgasm induced by tricyclic antidepressants, MAOIs, and antipsychotic agents.

Cautions

Refer to the General Statement regarding antihistamines. In general, however, the safety and efficacy of this drug has not been established for children under 2 years of age. There is no known evidence for carcinogenic or mutagenic activity. There is no known impairment of fertility or lactation in humans. It is unknown if cyproheptadine is concentrated in breast milk. For this reason caution should be exercised when this drug is administered to nursing women.

Dosage and Administration

Dosage. The administration of cyproheptadine should be adjusted to the individual's needs and tolerance. The usual initial dosage of cyproheptadine is 4 mg three times a day in adults. Many adults may require 12 to 16 mg/day. In general, dosage should not exceed 0.5 mg/kg/day. In the management of anorgasmia, 4 to 12 mg of cyproheptadine may be administered 1 to 2 hours before anticipated sexual activity or 1 to 8 mg may be administered on a daily basis.

Administration. Cyproheptadine is administered orally.

Preparations

Cyproheptadine hydrochloride
- Oral solution (*Periactin Syrup*)
  - 2 mg/5 mL
- Tablets (Periactin)
  - 4 mg

DIPHENHYDRAMINE

Pharmacokinetics

Absorption. Diphenhydramine is rapidly absorbed following oral administration and subsequently undergoes significant first-pass metabolism with approximately 40% to 60% of the oral dose

Table 9–1.
Drug Interactions With Antihistamines

Combination	Interaction	Mechanism/ Comment	Clinical Significance
Alcohol or other CNS depressants	↑ Sedative effects of all CNS depressants (↑ impairment of motor and mental performance)	Additive synergistic CNS depressant effect of each agent (?) Warn patients of danger of coadministration Wide variation among individuals in effect of this combination	Yes
Aminosalicylic acid (PAS) diphenhydramine	↓ Plasma levels of PAS	Diphenhydramine appears to impair GI absorption of PAS	?
Anticholinesterase agents, e.g., neostigmine, physostigmine	↓ Miotic effect by certain antihistamines which have significant anticholinergic effect	Antagonized by anticholinergic (atropine-like) effect of antihistamines Avoid this combination if possible, particularly in patients at special risk (e.g. glaucoma)	?
Anticonvulsant (e.g., phenytoin + chlorpheniramine (Chlor-Trimeton)	↑ Blood levels of phenytoin	Impairs phenytoin metabolism Use this combination with caution	?

		Stop chlorpheniramine if patient shows signs of drowsiness, ataxia, diplopia, tinnitus, or occipital headache with vomiting (possible phenytoin toxicity)	
Tricyclic antidepressant (TCAs)	Augment anticholingeric effects of TCAs	Probably additive effects at receptor sites Adverse effects usually minor In geriatric patients may precipitate urinary retention, acute glaucoma, or adynamic ileus	?
Diphenhydramine + temazepam	Stillbirth at term	Mechanism? One case report Avoid this combination during pregnancy Experiments in rabbits showed dangers of stillbirths or perinatal deaths.	?
MAOIs, (phenelzine) + cyproheptadine (Periactin)	Visual hallucination	Mechanism unknown Case report	?

(Continued.)

Table 9–1 (cont.).

Combination	Interaction	Mechanism/ Comment	Clinical Significance
Metyrapone (Metopirone) + cyproheptadine	pituitary-adrenal response to metyrapone	Mechanism: a reduction in adrenocorticotropin secretion expected after metyrapone administration. Cyproheptadine should be discontinued before or avoid its use when metyrapone is used for pituitary-adrenal axis assessment	Yes
Propranolol + Chlorpheniramine	Inhibit the β-blocking effect of propranolol and enhances its quinidine-like effect (i.e., ↓ conduction velocity and ↑ effective refractory period)	Theoretical consideration: it has not been reported in humans or animals	?
Warfarin+ diphenhydramine	Has little or no effect on anticoagulant response	No special precautions appear necessary	?

reaching the systemic circulation. Peak levels are achieved 1 to 3 hours after oral administration.

Distribution. Diphenhydramine appears to be widely distributed in body tissue and fluids. Its exact distribution, however, has not been fully determined. It does cross the placenta and is found in the fetus. Furthermore, it is found in breast milk, but the exact concentrations are unknown. The drug is approximately 85% bound to plasma proteins.

Elimination. Diphenhydramine is almost entirely metabolized prior to elimination. Diphenhydramine and its metabolites are principally excreted in the urine.

Uses

Diphenhydramine may be used as a hypnotic for sleep induction. It is also effective in the prevention and treatment of nausea, vomiting, and vertigo when these are associated with motion sickness. Diphenhydramine is helpful in treating neuroleptic-induced parkinsonism and, when administered parenterally, in treating acute dystonic reactions.

Cautions

See the General Statement regarding antihistamines. Children may be more likely to develop paradoxical agitation in response to diphenhydramine. Furthermore, the efficacy and utility of diphenhydramine has not been completely established in children younger than 12 years of age. Caution should be exercised when other sedative-hypnotics are given with diphenhydramine. Co-administration may potentiate the sedative and hypnotic effects. Likewise, patients should be cautioned about engaging in hazardous activities such as operating machinery or driving vehicles while under the influence of diphenhydramine.

Pregnancy, Fertility, and Lactation. There are suggestions but no clear evidence that the use of diphenhydramine during the first trimester may be associated with an increased risk of teratogenesis. Cleft palate, either alone or combined with other fetal abnormalities, may be more frequent in children exposed to diphenhydramine in utero. Diphenhydramine is found in human breast milk. For this reason caution should be exercised when the drug is administered to nursing women.

Dosage and Administration

Dosage. The usual adult dosage is 25 to 50 mg three to four times a day. This dosage is used for treatment of neuroleptic-induced parkinsonism and motion sickness. For sleep induction 50 mg is taken orally 20 to 30 minutes prior to sleep. Diphenhydramine 50 mg administered IM or IV may be used to treat acute dystonic reactions.

Administration. Diphenhydramine is usually administered orally, but, it may also be administered IM or IV.

Preparations

Diphenhydramine hydrochloride
- Oral capsules
  - 25 mg (*Benadryl, Benadryl 25, Kapseals, Genahist, Nordryl 25*)
  - 50 mg (*Benadryl Kapseals, Nordryl 50, Sleepinal Nighttime Sleep Aid*)
- Elixir (*Benadryl Elixir, Diphen Genahist Elixir, Hydramine Elixir*)
  - 12.5 mg/5 mL
- Tablets, film-coated (*Benadryl 25*)
  - 25 mg
- Parenteral injection
  - 10 mg/mL (*Benadryl, Benahist 10, Benoject-10, Nordryl, Wehdryl-10*)
  - 50 mg/mL (*Benadryl, Benahist 50, Benoject-50, Diphenacen-50, Hyrexin-50*)

INDEX

E

Q

R

S

T

U

V